"In the realm of self-improvement books, focusing on a single area, such as diet or happiness, is a very common construct. Much rarer (and typically less successful) is a volume that attempts to take a holistic approach to virtually every aspect of life. Chayne, a recent college graduate, not only manages to cover a great deal of territory, but she does it with authority…

The volume is remarkable in its ability to condense material of substance into bite-size segments. The benefit of this approach is significant: Chayne paints with a very broad brush, offering a taste of many issues both large and small in just enough detail to get one's mind working. In this respect, the book delivers an impressive format: an encyclopedic work in scope that has been adapted to contemporary environment for people who have neither the inclination nor the time to read a lot of specifics.

An elegantly written, passionately presented, cleverly organized guide to pursuing a healthy and responsible life."

—Kirkus Reviews

THRIVE

An Environmentally Conscious Lifestyle Guide

to Better Health and True Wealth

K. CHAYNE

ISBN-10: 0-997 1320-2-7
ISBN-13: 978-0-9971320-2-1

Purpose Prints
Konscious World
konscious.co

Disclaimer: This book is not intended to be a substitute for the medical advice of licensed physicians. The reader should consult with his/her doctors regarding any matters relating to his/her health and especially regarding any symptoms that may require diagnosis or medical attention.

Mention of specific people, companies, or organizations in this book does not imply endorsement by the author or the publisher, nor does it imply that the mentioned people, companies, or organizations endorse this book, its author, or the publisher.

Dedication

I dedicate this book to you.

To exist
is to be at one point in time.

To live
is to experience every passing moment
with your five senses and your mind open.

To Thrive
is to think beyond what is best for each of us right now
and to act upon what is best for our world for the future.

And *that* is the rarest thing of all.

It is our collective selflessness
that can give us a chance to create a *forever*.

—K. Chayne

Table of Contents

Opening

In chasing after our goals, many of us forget to open our minds and five senses to truly live in the moment. We also neglect our need to take care of our minds, bodies, and environment so we can thrive in the future. We may not be able to change the past, but we can begin to live our lives with a new sense of vigor, passion and purpose, starting right now.

Unfortunately, in today's world of supersonic speed, where we fill every minute of every day to capacity with activities, we leave little time to learn how to efficiently and effectively care for ourselves. But if you have picked up this book, you are in luck. I understand that your time is precious. Therefore, this book will not be an overwhelming encyclopedic guide, but an evidence-based summary of how you can begin to live a healthier, happier life right away.

Because of how much our environment affects us, a healthy decision is one that is not only beneficial to us but also to our environment. Therefore, we need to broaden our definition of "healthy" to encompass both direct and indirect health effects. After all, a healthier ecosystem—clean, fresh waters, unpolluted air, and diverse, nutritious sources of food—can ultimately sustain healthier species.

Of course, changing the way we live or view the world is much easier said than done. Where do we even begin? The start to any positive lifestyle change must begin first with *awareness* and *understanding*. Total wellness can be achieved only by having a healthy mind, body, and environment. Therefore, we must understand first how to build psychological resources, what each of our own bodies needs to thrive, and how our choices may affect the way our natural ecosystems function. With stronger mind-body-environmental connections, we will then be able to recraft our thought processes, habits and daily decisions to create sustainability in all areas of our lives.

After reading this book, you will have obtained practical, foundational knowledge on the following: how to be happy and influential through positive thinking; how to healthfully live by engaging in effective, regular physical activity and following holistically balanced diets; how to become a mindful shopper of eco-friendly and nontoxic products; and how to travel in ways that will transform you and the people you meet. Although not everything discussed in *Thrive* will be new to you, I hope the book in its entirety will inspire you to adopt a more holistic perspective on health—a perspective that is necessary for our survival, yet one that is often overlooked.

At this moment, please allow this to be not only the opening of this book, but also the opening of your mind. We often trap ourselves with *confirmation bias*, allowing new information into our minds only if it supports what we already believe. This can be extremely dangerous. It not only prevents us from true learning, but it also narrows our vision. It is only when we learn to welcome new challenges and embrace the ever-changing discoveries around us, that we are able to develop a solid, up-to-date understanding of ourselves and our world.

I sincerely hope that this book will encourage you to see how much you matter as an individual and will empower you to make more informed, healthy choices in life. And, above all, I hope it will inspire you to not only live, but *Thrive*.

Now, if you are ready, get excited to learn how to recraft your lifestyle from the inside out to better health, true wealth, and a better, healthier world!

PART I

SMILE

"There are flowers everywhere,
for those who bother to look."
—Henri Matisse

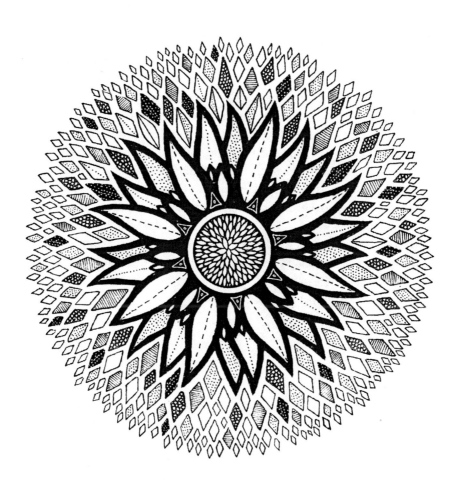

Chapter 1

Enter Your World Within

Happiness is something we all want in life, and we use the "pursuit of happiness" to guide our everyday desires and goals. We often make decisions because we feel that they will make us happy. However, those living life for the pursuit of happiness are in for a surprise: happiness is neither a destination nor something to conquer. There is no magic pair of shoes you can buy or city you can move to that will bring you an ultimate "happily ever after." Instead, happiness is an ongoing attitude and way of living that you take with you no matter where you go, what situations you encounter, or whom you meet in life.

One of the primary goals of this book is to help you realize and obtain "psychological wealth" (or "true wealth"). What does this mean? The wealth we often hear of refers to monetary riches, but *psychological wealth,* as defined by psychologists Ed Diener and Robert Biswas-Diener, includes "life satisfaction, the feeling that life is full of meaning, a sense of engagement in interesting activities, the pursuit of important goals, the experience of positive emotional feelings, and a sense of spirituality that connects people to things larger than themselves."[1] To live meaningfully and healthily, we need not only sufficient material resources for physical sustenance, but also spiritual, social, and psychological ones. Therefore, obtaining true wealth—*psychological* wealth—is crucial, because these are the riches we will need in life to be happy, to have motivation to pursue our passions and dreams, and also to rebound from the individual hardships that each of us will inevitably face in life.

Happiness usually includes three factors:

1. frequent positive feelings;

2. infrequent negative feelings; and

3. a global sense of satisfaction with life.[2]

Nevertheless, happiness can still mean "different things to different people," as that song goes. For example, there are even cultural differences in what happiness signifies. Asian cultures tend to view happiness as social harmony and a peacefully content mood, while Western cultures tend to view happiness as individually oriented and a more upbeat, exciting emotion.[3] Due to the varying ways in which people perceive happiness, in psychology, *happiness* is referred to as "subjective well-being," allowing room for personal interpretations. No matter—happiness is consistently seen by people of all origins and cultures as a desirable, pleasant emotional state.

It is certainly nice to feel good. However, there is much more to happiness than just being able to bask in a pleasant state of mind, because happiness is actually a functional asset that may affect all areas of our lives. A substantial amount of research has been conducted in recent years on *positive psychology*, which studies potential interventions that can help someone achieve life satisfaction. Generally speaking, happier people (typically determined by self-reporting measurements) tend to live longer, have fewer illnesses, stay married longer, commit fewer crimes, have more creative ideas, work harder, perform better at work, make more money, and help others more.[4] Thus, making a conscious effort to maintain and boost mental health is not only beneficial for feeling good right now but also for giving you the potential for a brighter future and a longer, happier life.

Although there are certain determinants of happiness that you cannot control, such as your genetic makeup and your life circumstances, the third factor of happiness—personal intentions—is completely in your hands. To help you boost your mental well-being, and to help you cultivate a sense of life satisfaction, the following chapters will guide you to:

- reshape your perspectives and thought processes;

- better cope with negative emotions and hardships;

- develop more psychological resources and meaningful relationships; and

- strengthen your connection to our world as a whole.

Enjoy the Ride

Why are there people who seemingly have everything—beautiful homes, successful careers, supportive families and friends, good physical health, etc.—but still live in frustration, trying to find happiness? On the other hand, why are there people living in poverty with joy? The answer is that happiness is neither a destination nor a single goal to be achieved. It is a process and way of living.

Think about it: We spend the majority of our lives within the "process" phases of different activities, and only ever-fleeting moments do we bask in the glory of accomplished goals. Therefore, learning to enjoy not only favorable outcomes, but also the entire journey along the way, can help us to gain long-term life satisfaction.

Let us examine the following different approaches to the same task. Two people, Pedro and Jenny, are collaborating on and completing a month-long science project to win an award. Unfortunately, in the end, they lose.

Pedro's approach: He focuses on the outcome, keeping his eye on the target. There is so much to do, and the process stresses him out. But it's okay, because he knows it will be worth it if they win. When Jenny cracks a joke while they work, Pedro becomes angry and tells her they cannot afford to lose time. He reminds himself constantly about the glory he would have and how proud his parents would be if they won the award. When they don't win, he is extremely upset and feels like the past month and his efforts were all wasted. He shamefully lowers his head in front of others, worrying that they might think of him as a failure.

Jenny's approach: Jenny knows what the goal is, but she also focuses on making the most of right now. She is stressed as well, but she views the project as a learning process and tries to make it enjoyable. After all, the project lets her spend more time with her friend. When they don't win, she is a little disappointed, but she is not brought down too hard. She tells herself that it definitely would have been a bonus if they had received an award for their hard work, but at least she learned a great deal from working on the project and really enjoyed the past month.

How is it that Pedro felt like he had *lost* so much, while Jenny felt like she had *gained* so much from working toward the same goal? The answer is: Pedro focused on only the results, while Jenny made the most of every moment throughout the process. Even if they had won the award, Jenny still would have gained more than Pedro had.

Every day, we constantly shift our thoughts from the past and the present to the future. However, we must use our unique abilities to do so to our advantage. Instead of being trapped in past failures and hardships, ask yourself how you can best *learn* from them. Instead of living for the future, savor the current moment and use your goals to guide your path. On your journey to accomplishing your dreams, don't forget to consciously look for the beautiful happenings around you and appreciate your moments in time.

Make Heaven of Hell

There are always multiple sides to a story. Consider the following event:

The facts: Two friends, Grumpy and Happy, go on vacation in Hawaii together for three days. They encounter terrible traffic on their way to the airport, but they still catch their flight just in time. When they finally get to Hawaii, it is pouring rain the first day and cloudy the next two days. Before heading back to the airport on their last day, they have breakfast outdoors when it is finally clear and sunny.

Grumpy's story: He complains about the traffic and blames Happy for not wanting to leave an extra half-hour early to avoid it. When they arrive in Hawaii and are greeted with heavy rain, Grumpy says that the day is a complete waste and they might as well have missed the flight. He also complains how "unlucky" they are when the next two days are cloudy. When it is finally sunny on the last day, he complains that the timing is horrible because they are about to leave.

Happy's story: He sits patiently through the traffic. If they miss their flight, he figures they can simply catch the next one. When they get to Hawaii, he shrugs off the unfortunate weather and instead runs into the pouring rain to get soaked for fun, because—well, why not? After all, they're in Hawaii! The next two days are cloudy, but he is happy because he still gets to enjoy the beach and go surfing. Finally, just before heading back to the airport, he feels thankful that he at least got a chance to witness the blue-skied paradise Hawaii is known for.

Same situation, two different people, two different perspectives, and two completely different experiences. This is the power of personal intentions! When you cannot change an undesirable outcome or situation, change your actions and outlook instead. John Milton, an English poet of the 17th century, famously said, "The mind is its own place, and in itself can make hell of heaven, or heaven of hell."

Going on vacation does not guarantee happiness if you focus on the inconveniences from traveling, the potentially rainy weather, and what you will miss while being away from home. Similarly, having a large salary does not guarantee happiness if you constantly compare yourself to others with even higher incomes and spend extravagantly in ways you cannot afford, in an effort to "keep up with the Joneses." As Sonja Lyubomirsky, author of *The How of Happiness* and professor of psychology at the University of California, Riverside, noted, "Happiness is not out there for us to find. The reason that it's not out there is that it's inside us."[5]

Steps to Positive Thinking

By nature, we get much more affected by undesirable events than by positive ones—a concept called *negativity bias*.[6] However, you can try to consciously combat this by choosing to magnify your blessings while downplaying or re-framing your misfortunes. To help you more effectively adopt positive attitudes, psychologists Ed Diener and Robert Biswas-Diener created the A.I.M. (attention, interpretation, and memory) intervention model.[7] As they discuss in their book, *Happiness: Unlocking the Mysteries of Psychological Wealth*, the three important steps to positive attitudes involve:

Attention

Because you are constantly bombarded with stimulation, you have to pick and choose what information your mind takes in. Therefore, positive thinking begins first with your becoming aware of the beautiful happenings around you. For example, when you socialize with others, think about what makes them great people instead of picking out their flaws.

Interpretation

There are always multiple ways of looking at a particular situation—some more positive, others more negative. However, you get to decide how you view the situation. If you catch yourself thinking negatively, *challenge* yourself to come up with a more positive interpretation of the same event. For example, if you catch yourself thinking that your friend left your house early because she thought you were boring, challenge that assumption. Maybe she left because she had some emergency at home, or because she remembered she had other personal errands to run. Or, if you catch yourself brooding over receiving a bad grade on an exam, translate that into motivation to learn from your mistakes and to do better in the future. Since you cannot change what already has happened, change your out-look and choose to see it as a learning process.

Alternatively, when you talk to yourself, implement the "Best Friend Tech-nique" developed by Richard Rakos (1991),[8] Associate Dean and Professor of Psychology at Cleveland State University. If you were to discuss your concerns with a best friend, how would your friend respond? Your friend is unlikely to agree with your negative interpretation of the situation but more likely to push you to see it in a different, more positive light.

Thankfully, reframing self-deprecating thoughts into more positive ones on your own is a skill that can be practiced and learned. It is like a muscle in your mind: the more you practice it, the more naturally it will come to you. At first, you might have to put some effort into practicing positive thinking. Eventually, however, your ability to refute your own negative thoughts will become a natural self-defense mechanism that can help boost your self-confidence and encourage you to see the world in a more positive manner.

Memory

Reminisce about the good times. When you have paid more *attention* to the good things and have learned to *interpret* situations more positively, you will have more positive *memories* to reflect upon afterward. Get into the habit of using Diener and Biswas-Diener's A.I.M. approach to positive thinking, and it will soon become a self-perpetuating, beneficial cycle.

Practice Gratitude—You'll Thank Me Later

Gratitude is an appreciative attitude toward one's blessings and a readiness to express gratefulness toward others. In recent years, extensive research has shown that consistent gratitude not only enhances one's personal well-being and relationships with others, but also makes one more energetic, forgiving, helpful, and satisfied with life.[9-12] Moreover, the positive effects of gratitude are not limited to the present moment. Practicing gratitude can actually lead to *sustained, long-term* levels of positivity.

Furthermore, having and expressing gratitude is beneficial to everyone involved. For example, when you have an appreciative attitude toward a friend, it will not only make him or her feel loved but also boost your own well-being and even strengthen your mutual relationship.[13] Gratitude is a positive mindset that creates even more positivity and goodwill in you and in others. Here are some ways you can practice gratitude:

- Keep a gratitude journal and jot down things you are thankful for a few times per week.

- Frequently express your appreciation to your family and friends.

- Write thank you notes to your teachers, doctors, trainers, and so on.

- Slip thank you notes to people you may not even know well but who still contribute to your personal life in some way: mail-deliverers, street-cleaners, janitors, gardeners, etc.

- Think about what your life would be like without something positive that is already in your life. This exercise is called *mental subtraction*—you compare yourself to a hypothetical you, a version of yourself that is worse off in some way.[14] Practicing mental subtraction will stop you from taking for granted those positive things you already have.

The secret to increasing and sustaining positivity through gratitude is to find a *variety* of ways to do so. We are innately drawn to novelty, so mix up how you thank the people around you or how you count your fortunes!

The Power of Perception

When trying to gain self-knowledge, we often compare ourselves to others. For example, knowing that you received an 84 on your exam does not provide you with much information on how you really performed. What if the average score was only 40? What if most people got over 90? To seek context, you are likely to resort to social comparisons.

When you compare yourself to people who are worse off than you (called *downward comparison*), you are likely to feel better about yourself. Meanwhile, when you compare yourself to people who are better off than you (called *upward comparison*), you might feel worse about yourself. However, studies have revealed that not all upward comparisons are equal and that what matters most is how you choose to see the comparison.[15, 16] For example, if you see someone better than you as superior to you, it will decrease your self-esteem and make you feel inferior. Meanwhile, if you see the same individual as an *inspiration* to you, it will enhance your perception of yourself and motivate you to improve. Therefore, regardless of your performance relative to others, just remember that *you* have control over how you perceive yourself and how you interpret the external information you obtain.

Chapter Summary

Enjoy the Ride

Happiness is not about having something at any one point in time but about a positive way of living all the time. Since we spend most of our lives in the "process" phases of our goals, remembering to make the most of the present can help us savor and enjoy our lives as much as possible.

Make Heaven of Hell

Although the first two determinants of happiness are uncontrollable (genetics and circumstances), the third factor, **personal intentions**, is completely in your hands. Therefore, by choosing to focus on the bright side of any given situation rather than to amplify the negatives, you will be able to live more positively and healthily.

Steps to Positive Thinking

Psychologists Ed Diener and Robert Biswas-Diener developed the **A.I.M.** model to guide you toward positive thinking. First, draw your **attention** toward the positive happenings around you, and try to **interpret** your circumstances in more favorable ways. You will thus have more pleasant **memories** to reminisce about.

Practice Gratitude; You'll Thank Me Later

Practicing **gratitude** has been consistently shown to enhance one's inner well-being. Not only will the people around you respect you more for your grateful attitude toward them and toward life in general, but you will also become happier and more satisfied with life.

The Power of Perception

We often compare ourselves to others to better understand our own performance relative to others. While downward comparisons will most likely boost our self-esteem, upward comparisons may make us feel inferior and hurt our self-confidence. However, we must remember the power of **perception** and use it to our advantage. Instead of seeing someone who performed better as being superior, think of that person as an inspiration instead.

Chapter 2

Break Down Bad

Emotions—joy, excitement, thrill, fear, anger, guilt—are what make us feel alive. But feelings are more than just feelings. They enhance our understandings of ourselves and of the people around us, and they also help us to regulate our behaviors. They keep us chasing after our dreams, but they also keep us away from potential threats and regrets.

As discussed in Chapter 1, positive moods actually serve a purpose. For example, they can help people boost their creativity, process information more effectively, and become more social. Over time, the positive consequences of happiness can help us build a sense of security, serving as mental resources to continually motivate us to cultivate meaningful relationships with others and pursue our passions. When things get rough, our psychological resources and feelings of security can also help us to better combat challenges and stress.

While being happy certainly has benefits, however, the ideal level of happiness is actually not being as happy as possible 100% of the time. In fact, extreme levels of happiness—characterized by heightened degrees of happiness and/or a relative absence of negative emotion—do not have health benefits and can even result in negative outcomes.[17] Instead, the ideal level of happiness is simply being mildly happy most of the time.

Strike a Healthy Balance

In life, there is simply no good without the bad and no bad without the good. While being happy is great, it is okay to be upset, too. Just as pleasant emotions are functional, so are negative ones. For example, feelings of guilt, anger, sadness, or fear help us to maintain our relationships with the outside world. Feeling sad after hurting a close friend will probably motivate you to mend your valued friendship, or fearing heights can keep you away from danger.

You need to be concerned about your negative emotions only when they begin to occur more often than your positive emotions do. Since it is unhealthy to be trapped inside of negativity for prolonged periods of time, if you ever catch yourself in this state, you will have to make more conscious effort than usual to combat and address your sources of negativity.

Find Stress Reducers That Fit *You*

Stress is that unpleasant feeling that seems to follow us everywhere. It is easy to simply give in to stress and accept it as it is. However, stress has been connected to all of the leading causes of death: heart disease, cancer, accidents, cirrhosis, suicide, etc.[18] Chronic stress can also accelerate the aging process.[19] Therefore, we must learn how to deal with stress to maintain mental and physical health and prevent chronic illnesses.

To find the most effective stress reducers for you, think about what activities you enjoy and how much free time you can regularly dedicate to them. (See also the section in Chapter 6 called, "Get Fit With Activities That Fit You.") For example, if you are extremely busy, it would not make sense for you to try to free up two hours every day to go to the gym. Instead, you can incorporate stress reducers that more easily fit into your established schedule, such as taking short stretch breaks every hour, chatting with friends during your lunch-breaks, listening to music on your commutes, and strolling around your neighborhood when you get home from work. It is all about finding the right set of activities that *fit* your personal lifestyle and interests.

Here are some examples of activities that help reduce stress:

- Walking through a park or green space

- Aerobic exercises (i.e., any exercise that increases your heart-rate to sustained levels at least 10 minutes at a time: running, speed-walking, cycling, swimming, etc.)

- Any physical activity that involves repetitive movements, requires rhythmic breathing, and is noncompetitive, predictable in nature, and not too intense (walking, moderate aerobic exercising, etc.)

- Low-impact, mindful activities (e.g., yoga)

- Meditation

- Getting some exposure to sunlight, indoors or outdoors

- Listening to calming music

- Getting a massage

- Socializing with friends and family

- Playing with a pet

- Painting, drawing, or writing, if you enjoy creative activities

- Writing about your Best Possible Self (see Chapter 3)

Beyond partaking in leisure activities to reduce your current stress level, you can also practice stress-preventing habits to minimize the amount of stress you might accumulate at a later point in time. Try to actively anticipate problems that might arise in the future by planning ahead accordingly. For example:

- Wake up 15 minutes earlier in the morning to prevent any morning mishaps or the need to rush your morning routine.

- Frequently practice preventative maintenance so your car and home appliances will be less likely to break down at an inconvenient time.

- Plan ahead and avoid procrastinating to prevent doing something "too late." If you think of something you need to do, complete the task right away, or immediately write down a reminder for its completion at a later time, but as soon as possible.

- Be flexible with change, be okay with imperfection, and be open-minded to novelty. If you accept the fact that things will not always go as planned, and instead learn to embrace whatever comes your way, life will be less stressful and more exciting!

Meditate Your Way to Good Health

Meditation may have religious or spiritual origins, but neurologists and psychologists have concluded from numerous research studies that meditation is actually beneficial to our health. For example, meditation has been shown to boost mood, decrease stress,[20,21] strengthen the immune system, aid various medical conditions, and improve psychological functions involving attention, compassion, and empathy.[22-24]

The beauty of meditation is that it is really for anyone and everyone, from the spiritual to the nonspiritual, from beginners to experts. It also does not require a lot of time and can be done whenever and wherever you like, making it a versatile activity suitable for any lifestyle. All you really need is a comfortable seat and some personal instructions to follow.

Michelle Jayne, an Australian yoga instructor who is also an avid practitioner of meditation (MichelleJayne.com.au), shares with us the following meditation guide that focuses on breathing. Since your eyes are supposed to be closed when you meditate, have someone read the guide to you or read it through once before you begin.

Meditation Guide

Close your eyes and turn your attention inward. Soften your forehead and relax your jaw; let go of the tension in your body as you surrender into a comfortable seated or lying position.

Bring your awareness to your abdomen and feel your belly rise as you inhale and soften as you exhale. As you inhale, feel the gradual expansion from your belly, to your ribcage, to your chest; and as you exhale, feel the gradual recession of your belly, then your ribcage, and then finally your chest.

Allow your mind to settle with the natural ebb and flow of your breaths. Notice that as the mind becomes quiet, your breathing becomes more balanced and complete.

As you breathe, notice any hidden tensions held in your breathing, body, or mind. As you exhale, let these pockets of tension melt away, one by one. Wherever you sense tension, simply relax when you exhale. While still being aware of your breathing, have the intention for your breathing to become completely effortless.

If you find that your mind wanders or your attention strays, draw your focus back to a single breath. A breath does not exist in the future or in the past. Thus, by drawing your awareness back to your breathing, you are being fully present in the moment.

As your mind settles, and your breathing becomes steady and effortless, know that in this moment of stillness, you are whole and complete. In this moment, you are exactly where you are meant to be.

When you are ready, start to deepen your breaths and make small movements with your hands and feet. Slowly begin to reconnect with the sensations of your surroundings, then open your eyes and come out of your meditation.

Forgive to Freedom

If someone hurt you, why forgive your offender? You may want to take revenge and make that person pay for it. But if you choose this route, *you* may be the one ultimately paying the price. Consider the following story:

The facts: Four best friends, Ann, Ben, Callie, and Daniel have been planning a farewell dinner for months. The dinner will be the last time they see one another before they split up to attend graduate schools in different cities. However, Daniel backs out at the last minute to go on a date with someone he barely knows, and he lies to Ann, Ben, and Callie, telling them he caught the flu. His friends find out about his lie when they coincidentally run into him in the town plaza after dinner.

Ann's reaction (revenge): She is furious that Daniel lied to them, as they have all been best friends ever since they were little. She feels that Daniel undermined their friendship, and that he deserves to pay for being untruthful. She schemes over the next two weeks on how to hurt him back.

Ben's reaction (conditional forgiveness): He is extremely sad and feels undervalued as a best friend to Daniel. He knows that Daniel did not mean to hurt him, but he waits in frustration over the next two weeks, wondering when he will receive a sincere apology from Daniel. He loses his appetite and is unable to focus in school.

Callie's reaction (unconditional forgiveness): Like Ann and Ben, she is hurt by Daniel's lie, as they all made a pact years ago to always be truthful to one another. However, even before receiving an apology, Callie calls Daniel to forgive him despite her disappointment in him. She is honest with him, though, and tells him that it will take some time for their friendship to return to the way it was. Over the next few weeks, Daniel's lie barely crosses Callie's mind, and Callie is able to socialize and work productively at school.

Daniel's reaction: Daniel is extremely ashamed of what he did, and he is unsure of how to make it up to his friends. When he gets home that night, he receives the unfortunate news that his aunt passed away. Over the next few weeks, he is preoccupied with planning his aunt's memorial service, contacting his professors at graduate school, rearranging his travel plans, and consoling his family members. When Callie calls to forgive him, he is touched and pleasantly surprised by her reaction. He is then inspired and determined to become a better friend to all of his peers.

Which reaction led to the best outcome? While the unforgiving Ann and Ben spent most of their following weeks being upset over the situation, the forgiving Callie was able to free herself and move on. Her forgiveness also inspired Daniel to become a better friend in the future.

When someone wrongs you, you have three general options:

1. to take revenge;

2. to wait for the transgressor's apology (*conditional forgiveness*); or

3. to begin to forgive within your own mind, regardless of whether the transgressor has apologized (*unconditional forgiveness*).

Since bearing grudges harbors negative emotions, planning a payback or waiting on an apology can both potentially contribute to adverse health effects by perpetuating anger and elevating your blood pressure.[25] And, even though conditional forgiveness involves forgiving, it still keeps people trapped in resentment and has been associated with higher risks for mortality from all causes.[26]

Thus, it is in your best interest to practice unconditional forgiveness when someone hurts you; doing so will not only make you the "bigger person" in the picture, but can also free you from being trapped inside of the distressing situation. As Siddhartha Gautama said, "Holding on to anger is like grasping a hot coal with the intent of throwing it at someone else; you are the one getting burned."

You do not necessarily need to restore your relationship with the individual who harmed you, but think about the power of forgiveness, not only to free yourself from negativity, but also to inspire the people around you, even the person who offended you. After all, forgiveness can disrupt that "eye-for-an-eye, tooth-for-a-tooth" mentality and give you an open door to move on through.

Find Meaning in Adversity

Sometimes, life is tough, and we all inevitably face hardships in varying degrees at different stages of our lives. While it may not be so difficult to look for the beautiful things in our lives and appreciate them, learning to find meaning in adversity can be more of a challenge.

As one might predict, higher incidences of adversity (illness, a loved-one's illness, violence, bereavement, social or environmental stress, relationship stress, natural disasters, etc.) are associated with higher levels of distress, functional impairment, post-traumatic symptoms, and lower life satisfaction.[27] However, this relationship is not linear. Adversity does not always make one less happy over the long run, as people with histories of *some* lifetime adversity were found to have *higher* levels of life satisfaction and resilience than those who faced no hardships at all.[28]

This finding supports the common saying, "What does not kill you can make you stronger." Hardships not only teach us to better cope with challenges, but also boost our confidence in our abilities to handle tough situations in the future. Not that we should celebrate misfortunes, but that "people are not doomed to be damaged by adversity," and dealing with hardships can help us to develop stronger levels of resilience.[29]

Although there is no definite path you must take to overcome your challenges, there are certain things you can do to facilitate your efforts to do so. For example:

- Write about the experience and about how you feel. This will help you to reflect upon the unpleasant event in a calm manner at a later time.

- First, tell yourself, "It will be okay," even if you are still upset. Then come up with as many reasons as possible for *why* it will be okay. This forces you to strengthen your self-defense mechanism and focus on the positives of the situation, no matter how trivial they may be.

- Use the "Best Friend Technique" (discussed in Chapter 1) to push yourself to see the situation more favorably.

- Surround yourself with loving, upbeat peers as much as possible, and open yourself up to allow their positivity to rub off on you.

- Remind yourself that when you come out on the other side, you will be stronger, more resilient, and more self-confident.

- Practice meditation or other stress-reducing strategies.

When in self-doubt, think upon these wise words of Andrew Solomon, a writer on politics, culture, and psychology, from his TED Talk, "How the Worst Moments in Our Lives Make Us Who We Are."

> We don't seek the painful experiences that hew our identities, but we seek our identities in the wake of painful experiences. We cannot bear a pointless tor-

ment, but we can endure great pain if we believe that it's purposeful. Ease makes less of an impression on us than struggle. We could have been ourselves without our delights, but not without the misfortunes that drive our search for meaning. [30]

Chapter Summary

Strike a Healthy Balance

Negative emotions, just like positive emotions, are functional. They help us to regulate our behaviors and maintain our relationships with the outside world. So, as long as your negative emotions don't take over your neutral and positive ones, don't be upset about being upset. Instead, find the reasons behind your negative emotions and try to address their root causes.

Find Stress Reducers That Fit You

Because stress affects our health in so many ways and can lead to chronic lifestyle diseases, we must develop our own unique ways to cope with our frustrations. To effectively reduce stress, come up with your own personal set of stress reducers that fit your interests and lifestyle. Also, try to plan ahead and practice stress-preventing habits that will minimize the chances of something unpleasant happening at the worst possible time.

Meditate Your Way to Good Health

Meditation may have spiritual origins, but it has been scientifically proven to boost mental and physical well-being. Fortunately, because there are so many variations of meditation that, for the most part, can be practiced anywhere at any time, you should be able to easily incorporate the practice into your regular routine.

Forgive to Freedom

Being wronged by someone can make you want to take revenge or ask for a heartfelt apology. However, try practicing **unconditional forgiveness**. That is, try to forgive your transgressor whether or not he or she has already apologized. This does not mean you have to become friendly with your transgressor. However, instead of being trapped in negativity, unconditional forgiveness can help you to move on faster, make you the bigger person in the situation, and even inspire your transgressor and others around you to become better people.

Chapter Summary (Cont'd)

Find Meaning in Adversity

We all face challenges in our lives at various times, and at various levels of intensities and durations. When you do, try to make sense of your situation and think about what you can learn from it. Finding meaning in adversity will not be easy, but when you come out on the other side, you will be stronger, more self-confident, and better able to cope with future challenges.

Chapter 3

Build Meaningful Riches

Recrafting your life to better health and true wealth will require long-lasting lifestyle changes: adopting healthier mentalities, instilling healthier habits into your daily regimen, and making healthier decisions. However, to actually translate your motivations into action and to bring about long-term lifestyle changes will take time and conscious effort. Even if you are ready to live life with a renewed sense of vigor and passion, you will not wake up tomorrow automatically a different person. However, the more conscious effort you put in, the more quickly you will develop a lasting positive attitude, the more likely your sustainable habits and choices will stick, and the healthier you will become overall.

Take Control

The first and arguably most important step in changing a habit is *awareness*. For example, if you do not even realize that you frequently criticize others, how can you begin to be less critical? To gain self-awareness, you will have to practice *introspection*. Think about why you do what you do, what motivates you to say what you say, and what stimulates you to react the way you react. If you are upset, think about the root causes of this emotion. Has someone seriously wronged you? Is it situational? Or is it merely from built-up stress? Will displacing your anger onto others make anything better? Or will it just damage your relationships with your loved ones? *Pause* for a few seconds before you act or say something aloud, and think about your motivations and the potential consequences of what you might say or do.

Once you become more self-aware, you can then use the following A.B.C. model (Antecedents, Behaviors, Consequences) from behavioral psychology to deter unwanted thoughts and behaviors and to encourage healthier ones.[31]

Antecedents

The *antecedents* to your behavior are the events that trigger your response. The purpose of isolating the cues to your behavior is to help you set up new antecedents that encourage healthier behaviors while discouraging less healthy ones.

If you frequently bite your nails in response to stress, stress would be the *antecedent* to your unwanted behavior. Here, you can find alternative ways to handle stress, and also set up an environment that deters your nail-biting behavior. For example, you can paint your nails, make little pencil marks on them, or wear gloves so it will make you think twice before starting that old habit again. Or, if your goal is healthier eating, you can begin by planning to eat at restaurants that offer only healthy choices; throwing out junk food from your cabinets at home; or dining with friends who are already health-conscious.

Behaviors

Think about what behaviors or thoughts you want to modify and what you would want to replace them with. Observe and model after people who are really good at the habits you want to adopt, and mimic their behaviors. For example, if your goal is to go to the gym more often, examine how your athletic friends motivate themselves to go, spend more time with them, and tell them to invite you to join them the next time they visit the gym.

Consequences

The *consequences* are the results of your behavior—what happens immediately after you do or say something. Set up self-regulation systems that reward your healthy behaviors, or discourage your unhealthy behaviors after you perform them. There is no right or wrong way to do this; it depends on personal preference. However, one easy way you can self-regulate is to set up a point system. For example, you can give yourself a point every time you choose to walk or bike somewhere instead of drive. Then, after you accumulate ten points, you can reward yourself with an hour of free time dedicated to an activity you enjoy. Alternatively, any time you conduct an unwanted behavior, you can take away points or time dedicated to leisure activities.

When you think of rewards, for the most part, avoid ones that revolve around consumption (food or material goods) except for the occasional treat or special occasion. Instead, focus on rewards that involve gaining positive experiences. If setting up your own consequences proves to be difficult, involve your family or close friends to assist you with the process.

When you first begin to instill healthier habits, keep your changes small (i.e., break big changes down into smaller, step-by-step changes), and don't feel guilty if you make mistakes or relapse—this is perfectly natural during a learning process. However, by giving your mind and body plenty of time to adjust to your lifestyle changes, your new set of habits will be more likely to stay for the long-term.

Do What You Love, Love What You Do

What activities do you get excited about? What are some of your hobbies? Engaging in enjoyable activities on a regular basis is extremely important in maintaining and improving mental health. Indeed, research has shown that sustained increases in happiness can be more easily achieved through changing what you *do* rather than changing your circumstances.[32] As Lyubomirsky noted, "There is no happiness without action."[33] Get into the habit of doing something you enjoy every day and building those activities into your routines.

Of course, we cannot always decide what we do, what our jobs are, or what our employers ask of us. No matter—we can still learn to appreciate our daily routines more using the power of perception.

From a psychological standpoint, there are three ways of looking at a job.[34,35] What type of attitude do you have toward yours? (See Table 3-1)

Table 3-1. Three Ways of Looking at a Job[36]

Orientation	How I Feel About My Job
Job Orientation	I see my job purely as a way to get money. I arrive to work at the last minute possible, and I look forward to getting off every day.
Career Orientation	I enjoy some parts of my job but not all. Ultimately, I see my job as a stepping-stone to future employment.
Calling Orientation	I would do this job even if I were not paid for it. I am passionate about it, and even do extra things not asked of me, simply because I enjoy doing so.

As you would have expected, people in the "Calling Orientation" have the highest levels of satisfaction at work and believe that what they do is fulfilling. To some extent, certain jobs may simply be more interesting or more impactful. However, one-third of workers in any given occupation consider their jobs to be a calling for them.[37] This suggests that it is not the job itself that determines whether it will be just a job, a career, or a calling to someone, but rather an individual's fit or perspective toward the job.

To further illustrate the power of personal interpretations, a study found that, while some hospital janitors viewed cleaning hospitals as a low-level job and disliked cleaning, others saw their roles as significant and contributive to the hospital community.[38] These calling-orientation cleaners saw their work as *integral* to the community's welfare, as they believed they were bettering the daily lives of the doctors, nurses, and patients by maintaining good hygiene in the hospital. They also frequently socialized with others within the community, were interested in finding new ways to do their jobs more efficiently, and even went out of their way to do tasks not asked of them.

Although most of us do not get to travel to exotic places, critique gourmet food, host fun social events, or make music for a living, we can all gain more satisfaction at work by altering our perspectives toward what we do. Think about how your role fits in as an integral part of a larger whole; think about the ways you impact your company or the people you work with; and think about how you can make your mandatory or mundane tasks more interesting.

When you have the choice, yes, choose to do what you love. However, when you are stuck with something, learn to love what you do. When future opportunities arrive for advancement or change, you can focus then on making the most of those opportunities and where they might take you.

Make a Living Out of Giving

It is not hard to be a member of a community or to make friends, but are your relationships meaningful to you? Fulfilling relationships involve continual reciprocity, compassion, and respect for one another. This means that you not only receive social support from your friends and family, but also commit to being there for them, which includes:

- actively dedicating time and thoughts to them;

- giving them hugs, which can make both of you happier and healthier;[39]

- being there for them when they are upset;

- basking in their glories with them, instead of envying them when they accomplish great feats;

- keeping their secrets;

- standing up for them;

- showing them that you appreciate them; and

- reciprocating their compassion.

In fact, *giving* support may be even more beneficial to one's health than *receiving* support. A study found that people who gave more to loved ones and neighbors lived longer than those who gave less, even after taking into account other potential factors, such as everyone's initial health conditions.[40] So, *live to give, and give to live!*

In the two-way street of relationships, we all affect our peers just as they affect each of us. Thus, surrounding yourself with positive, thoughtful friends may push you to see the world in a better light. On the other hand, being around chronic worriers may make you more anxious than you were before. To build a solid support system, find a healthy balance for yourself where you can positively impact your more pessimistic or anxious friends while allowing yourself to be motivated by your more upbeat peers.

To take giving to another level, you can also become a compassionate community member and world citizen. Volunteer in your local community, give your seat up to the elderly or disabled, express your appreciation toward your community members, hold the door open for people behind you, donate to charity, help the needy, support social and environmental causes, and so on. Your thoughtful, selfless behaviors will not only make your community a friendlier place, but also boost your mental well-being and strengthen your connection to a world larger than yourself.

The magical thing about giving is that it creates virtuous cycles that are integral to a thriving community. It really is a win-win situation for all, because such acts of kindness can have rippling effects throughout a community. When people witness others doing good things, they are more likely to conduct an act of altruism themselves.[41] Therefore, if you initiate ten acts of kindness throughout your day, you can expect that at least some of those recipients or witnesses of your kindness will continue to pass good deeds along.

Be that change you want to see in the world, and initiate acts of kindness that will ripple off into your neighborhoods, communities, and perhaps cities. Over time, you might even make an entire community a friendlier place without realizing it.

Envision to Know Your Mission

One of the most important ingredients to living a fulfilling life is to have a purpose. However, a purpose must be developed over time; it is not something you can sit down right now to come up with. In creating a purpose, it helps to begin by setting short-term goals for yourself.

An exercise associated with boosting subjective well-being is the Best Possible Self Exercise.[42] Take five minutes now and follow these adapted guidelines:

Best Possible Self Exercise

1. Pick a time in the future (one year or five years ahead) and visualize your Best Possible Self at that time. Visualize the best possible circumstances for you as they involve your friends, family, career, wealth, health, etc., in a way that highly satisfies and excites you.

2. Visualize the details vividly. Keep in mind that the successes you envision for yourself should be optimistic but realistic.

3. When you have a clear picture in mind of a best possible future version of you, write down the details on a piece of paper for a minute. Or simply hold on to that image in your head.

By now you should already be basking in a more positive mood than you were in previously. To push yourself another step further and transform your vision into goals you can actively work toward, do the following:

4. Think about what attitudes and character strengths you will need in order to achieve that best possible self. If you envision yourself as superpopular and well liked by your peers, a goal could be to become more *social* toward, and *considerate* of, the people around you. If you envision yourself as really successful with a new business, character strengths to focus on might include *creativity* and *perseverance*.

Architect Your Life Toward Meaning

The point in time when you realize your own purpose in life will be different from anyone else's. Maybe you already knew your purpose from a young age, or maybe you still have no idea. Regardless of what stage in life you are in, don't stress out if you feel lost, because every day you are one step closer to realizing what you really want out of life. Try things you never thought of trying before, befriend people who are very different from you, or travel to someplace you never thought you would go. After all, uncertainty is what makes life truly exciting and worth living. Every new day comes with opportunities for new discoveries if we only open ourselves up to them. Over time, all of these little experiences accumulate to shape what we know and who we are, as well as what we want out of life.

Needless to say, everyone's life journey is unique. Sometimes you merely need to start painting on a blank canvas without any idea of what you are trying to portray, or sometimes you already have a vivid sketch in mind. If you already have long-term goals, break them down into short-term plans so you can more easily transform your dream into reality. If you have no idea where you are going, pursue your short-term passions and become the architect of your life, building it from the bottom-up. Over time, without your even realizing it, all of your little strokes on the canvas will add up and lead you to a better picture of what you want your masterpiece to look like.

On your path toward crafting a purposeful life, it certainly helps to have goals for yourself. But how do you identify goals that can contribute to life satisfaction? The four areas in which people most likely search for meaning when building a fulfilling life are:

1. The *life-work dimension*, where you feel committed to your work and feel that what you do is engaging and meaningful (think job, career, calling, and regular participation in engaging activities).

2. The *relationship* dimension, where you develop valuable relationships and intimacy with other people based on mutual compassion, altruism, and reciprocity.

3. The *social* dimension, where you think and act beyond your personal self-interests to leave a legacy and an imprint on society.

4. The *spiritual* dimension, where you cultivate a deep connection to a certain religion, community of faith, the natural world, or something larger than yourself.[43,44]

When coming up with goals for yourself, whether short-term or long-term, make sure to address each of these life categories so you can most effectively create meaning out of your life!

Chapter Summary

Take Control

It is no simple task to recraft your thought processes, habits, and decisions. However, you can start by using the A.B.C. model. By first setting up helpful **antecedents** that will facilitate healthier **behaviors** (or thoughts), and then using rewarding **consequences** to further encourage the wanted behaviors, you will more easily adopt lasting lifestyle changes.

Do What You Love, Love What You Do

Happiness is about doing rather than having. So, get into the habit of doing something you enjoy every day. Although you may not get to decide what you do for a living, you can still make your job feel more satisfying by focusing on how you impact the people around you and how you fit into your work community as an integral part of a whole. When you have the option, choose to do what you love. However, when you are stuck with something, you might as well try to love what you do.

Make a Living Out of Giving

To cultivate meaningful relationships, you will have to become a **giver**. Actively dedicate time and thoughts to your loved ones, show them you appreciate them, reciprocate kind deeds, be there for them, celebrate their successes with them, and be loyal to them. Whenever you can, participate in altruistic behaviors within your local community, as witnessing an act of kindness influences others to be altruistic, too, and your kind deeds will benefit not only the recipients and you, but also your community at large.

Envision to Know Your Mission

To boost sustained levels of positivity, try the Best Possible Self Exercise, where you envision your best possible future self and then transform your vision into actionable short-term goals. The exercise will not only make you feel good, but also motivate you to translate your vision into reality.

Chapter Summary (Cont'd)

Architect Your Life Toward Meaning

We all want to live "meaningfully," but this will not happen overnight. It will take years of self-development and life experiences. If you have already discovered your purpose in life, break it down into smaller, actionable goals so you can transform your dream into reality. If you have no idea what life means to you, don't fret; just begin to architect your life from the bottom-up. Continue to explore new places, do what you enjoy, meet new people, obtain novel life experiences, and set short-term goals for yourself. With every day that passes, you will only get closer to your time of revelation.

Chapter 4

Call the World Home

As human beings, we tend to break down and categorize everything, giving things labels and drawing boundaries. While there are certainly benefits to this, it also narrows our perspectives and disconnects us from our world.

When considering the word *home,* people begin by thinking about their bedrooms, houses, neighborhoods, towns, cities and, finally, countries. Therefore, people end up being most protective of their houses, and then their neighborhoods, cities, countries, and so on. Where does this leave our planet as one's home?

Last.

Well, let us embrace our animal instincts for a second. As living creatures, what do we need in order to survive and thrive? We need diverse, nutritious sources of food, sunlight, clean air, and clean water—things only nature can give us. Unfortunately, nature knows no boundaries. Damages in another city's ecosystem, or even another continent's, will only do us all harm. Polluted rivers from another city can flow through ours and pollute our drinking water. Increases in greenhouse gas emissions from any factory in the world contribute to global climate change. Therefore, to cultivate healthy mindsets—ones that recognize the importance of our planet's holistic well-being—we must strengthen our connections to our world, see the importance of protecting our home planet as a whole, and reshape our thought processes, habits and decisions accordingly.

Science Says We Need Nature

Biophilia is Edward O. Wilson's theory from 1984 that humans have an innate need to affiliate with nature and other living species.[45] Since Wilson published his theory, research has suggested that exposure to natural landscapes can indeed be helpful in reducing stress, increasing productivity, and even improving physical health. For example, *nature connectedness,* which involves "a sense of meaningful involvement in something larger than oneself," has been shown to correlate positively with psychological and social well-being.[46-48] That is, people who are more connected to nature tend to be happier. If nature relatedness can be good not only for us but also our planet (because we would value and protect our planet more), cultivating stronger mind-body-environmental connections could be vital to both our personal health and our environment's sustainability.

Here are some other interesting findings related to biophilia:

- People reported and showed physiological signs of reduced stress levels after connecting with nature.[49]

- The presence of indoor plants correlated positively with the productivity of workers. It also reduced negative moods and levels of stress among building occupants.[50]

- Patients with rooms looking out into nature recovered faster than patients with rooms looking out onto brick walls.[51]

- A review of 50 empirical studies on biophilia concluded, "Even in individuals who do not express any appreciation for plants and nature, the lack of [exposure to] nature can have a negative effect."[52]

- Students with more natural views from their dormitory windows had better attention spans than those with less natural views.[53]

- According to a systematic review of nature-assisted therapy, "significant improvements were found for varied outcomes in diverse diagnoses, spanning from obesity to schizophrenia," and nature can be an important resource for mental and public health care.[54]

Furthermore, exposures to natural sunlight can rapidly increase one's level of serotonin, a neurotransmitter within our bodies that contributes to feelings of happiness.[55,56] Apparently, you can boost your mood simply by being outdoors when the sun is out! This probably does not come as a surprise to you—we often have the urge to be outside when it is sunny. Well, it turns out that good weather is nice for not only unfiltered Instagram photos, but also for your happiness!

So, get your daily dose of nature. Go outside and take a walk in the park. Stroll down a sidewalk filled with trees and shrubs. Plant a mini-garden in your backyard, on your balcony, or on your rooftop. Alternatively, you can try to bring the outdoors in as well. For example, you can open up your curtains during the daytime to let in natural sunlight, or decorate your interiors with some indoor plants (see also the section in Chapter 22 called, "An Eco-Sanctuary"). They not only can improve your indoor air quality but also might help you reduce stress and make you more productive!

Bigger, Broader, and Better

All of the boundaries we have drawn have merely led us to narrower visions and more isolated selves. For optimum health, however, we must develop broader perspectives and deepen our relationships to the home we all inhabit. To summarize, strengthening our connection with nature can have the following direct and indirect benefits:

- Psychological health benefits from connecting to a world greater than ourselves

- General health benefits from direct exposure to nature and sunlight

- Ecosystem health benefits from people striving to protect nature more

- Public health benefits from living on a healthier planet

In 2011, the Nature Conservancy conducted a poll of 602 children between ages 13 and 17 and found that children who reported having meaningful experiences in nature were more likely to appreciate outdoor activities and express concerns for environmental issues.[57] Perhaps urbanization has undermined our instincts to protect our natural resources. In our modern world, many of us lead lives within concrete landscapes—away from the lands that produce our food and away from the rivers and lakes that supply our drinking water. Many children today also grow up watching their meals magically appear at restaurants and their drinking water magically flow out of kitchen faucets. If we don't understand how our food is produced or how our water cycles through natural ecosystems, how will we come to appreciate and recognize the importance of protecting our planet?

The disconnect between people and nature, if left unaddressed, leads to ignorant behaviors that can be self-destructive without our even realizing it. Therefore, to understand how natural ecosystems function, to appreciate the necessities of life nature gives us, and to understand how our daily choices impact our planet are essential parts of a true, healthy mind.

Recraft Your Mindset

In our much-globalized world, you may feel very miniscule, and your actions and words perhaps insignificant. However, look at it in another way: Because everything is interconnected in our modern world, *everything* you do and say matters. You may not feel it, but you are impactful, and it is up to you to combine your knowledge and power into a driving force of good.

Negativity may be a vicious cycle, but positivity can be a *virtuous cycle*. When you are a loyal and caring friend, partner and family member, you are building for yourself a strong support system. When you partake in altruistic behaviors in your community, you will inspire others to do the same and make your community a better place to live. When you choose to be the bigger person in an unfair situation and resort to forgiveness rather than revenge and hatred, you will have ended a vicious cycle and opened new doors to a brighter future.

On your path to happiness, I hope you will see that building psychological wealth is best accomplished when you become the best person you can be. You may not be able to control what happens to you or how others treat you, but do not let misfortune or injustice define you. For you can get the best reflection of yourself by examining what *you* say and what *you* do.

I end this chapter by hoping to leave you thoughtfully ruminating on the importance of a healthy mindset—one that values your connection with nature—for a very important reason. As the book progresses, you will see how your daily decisions, even ones as mundane as what you choose to eat for lunch or which shirt you choose to buy, can impact our world in a good or bad way, thus impacting *you* in a good or bad way.

More importantly, you will see that choices beneficial for the health of our planet coincidentally are the choices better for *your* health as well. To thrive, our world requires biodiversity, uncontaminated waters, unpolluted air, and natural sunlight. To threaten any of these through our daily decisions is self-destructive, as the laws that govern our planet's health are the exact same ones that govern our own individual health. Therefore, I encourage you to broaden your definition of "healthy" and recraft your mindset to see that your health depends on our planet, and that our planet's health depends on you.

Chapter Summary

Science Says We Need Nature

Numerous studies support the theory of **biophilia,** which states we have an innate need to connect with nature. In fact, exposure to natural landscapes and sunlight has been shown to benefit both our mental and physical health. So, get your daily dose of greenery and natural daylight by visiting parks, strolling down tree-filled streets, planting your own private garden, or even accessorizing your home or office spaces with indoor plants.

Bigger, Broader, and Better

For optimum health, we need to **broaden** our perspectives and **deepen** our relationships to our planet. Especially at a time when we have become so disconnected from our world as a whole, getting in touch with nature can benefit not only our personal well-being but also our planet's sustainability.

Recraft Your Mindset

Although each of us is such a miniscule part of our planet, the impacts from our daily decisions have a ripple effect on our communities, countries, continents, and even our world. Therefore, focusing on reshaping your individual thoughts, habits, and daily decisions can have much more of an influence than you might think. Because of how our minds, bodies, and natural environment all impact one another, understanding how to efficiently and effectively care for yourself as well as our planet's ecosystem is a crucial step toward achieving holistic wellness.

Part References

1   Diener, E., & Biswas-Diener, R. (2008). *Happiness: Unlocking the mysteries of psychological wealth*. Malden, MA: Blackwell Pub.

2   Myers, D. G., & Diener, E. (1995). Who is happy? *Psychological Science, 6*(1), 10-19.

3   Lu, L., & Gilmour, R. (2004). Culture and conceptions of happiness: Individual oriented and social oriented SWB. *Journal of Happiness Studies, 5*(3), 269-291.

4   Diener, E., & Biswas-Diener, R. (2008). *Happiness: Unlocking the mysteries of psychological wealth*. Malden, MA: Blackwell Pub.

5   Lyubomirsky, S. (2008). *The how of happiness: A new approach to getting the life you want*. New York: Penguin Press, p40.

6   Baumeister, R., Bratslavsky, E., Vohs, K., & Finkenauer, C. (2001). Bad is stronger than good. *Review of General Psychology, 5*(4), 323-370.

7   Diener, E., & Biswas-Diener, R. (2008). *Happiness: Unlocking the mysteries of psychological wealth*. Malden, MA: Blackwell Pub.

8   Watson, D. L., & Tharp, R. G. (2013). *Self-directed behavior: Self-modification for personal adjustment* (10th ed.). Belmont, CA: Wadsworth Publishing.

9   Dusen, J. P., Tiamiyu, M. F., Kashdan, T. B., & Elhai, J. D. (2015). Gratitude, depression and PTSD: Assessment of structural relationships. *Psychiatry Research, 230*(3), 867-870.

10   Emmons, R. A., & McCullough, M. E. (2003). Counting blessings versus burdens: An experimental investigation of gratitude and subjective well-being in daily life. *Journal of Personality & Social Psychology, 84*(2), 377-389.

11   Froh, J., Miller, D., & Snyder, S. (2007). Gratitude in children and adolescents: Development, assessment, and school-based intervention. *School Psychology Forum*, 1-13.

12   Lyubomirsky, S. (2008). *The how of happiness: A new approach to getting the life you want*. New York: Penguin Press, p40.

13   Lambert, N. M., Clark, M. S., Durtschi, J., Fincham, F. D., & Graham, S. M. (2010). Benefits of expressing gratitude: Expressing gratitude to a partner changes one's view of the relationship. *Psychological Science, 21*(4), 574-580.

14 Koo, M., Algoe, S. B., Wilson, T. D., & Gilbert, D. T. (2008). It's a wonderful life: Mentally subtracting positive events improves people's affective states, contrary to their affective forecasts. *Journal of Personality and Social Psychology, 95*(5), 1217-1224.

15 Burleson, K., Leach, C. W., & Harrington, D. M. (2005). Upward social comparison and self-concept: Inspiration and inferiority among art students in an advanced programme. *British Journal of Social Psychology, 44*(1), 109-123.

16 Collins, R. L. (1996). For better or worse: The impact of upward social comparison on self-evaluations. *Psychological Bulletin, 119*(1), 51-69.

17 Gruber, J., Mauss, I. B., & Tamir, M. (2011). A dark side of happiness? How, when, and why happiness is not always good. *Perspectives on Psychological Science, 6*(3), 222-233.

18 Seaward, B. L. (2013). *Managing stress: Principles and strategies for health and well-being.* Sudbury, MA: Jones and Bartlett.

19 Epel, E. S., Blackburn, E. H., Lin, J., Dhabhar, F. S., Adler, N. E., Morrow, J. D., & Cawthon, R. M. (2004). Accelerated telomere shortening in response to life stress. *Proceedings of the National Academy of Sciences, 101*(49), 17312-17315.

20 Astin, J. A. (1997). Stress reduction through mindfulness meditation. *Psychotherapy and Psychosomatics, 66*(2), 97-106.

21 Miller, J. J., Fletcher, K., & Kabat-Zinn, J. (1995). Three-year follow-up and clinical implications of a mindfulness meditation-based stress reduction intervention in the treatment of anxiety disorders. *General Hospital Psychiatry, 17*(3), 192-200.

22 Hanson, R., & Mendius, R. (2009). *Buddha's brain: The practical neuroscience of happiness, love & wisdom.* Oakland, CA: New Harbinger Publications, p84.

23 Hölzel, B. K., Carmody, J., Vangel, M., Congleton, C., Yerramsetti, S. M., Gard, T., & Lazar, S. W. (2011). Mindfulness practice leads to increases in regional brain gray matter density. *Psychiatry Research: Neuroimaging, 191*(1), 36-43

24 Lyubomirsky, S. (2008). *The how of happiness: A new approach to getting the life you want.* New York: Penguin Press, p40.

25 van Oyen Witvliet, C., Ludwig, T. E., Vander Laan, K. L. (2001) Granting forgiveness or harboring grudges: implications for emotion, physiology, and health. *Psychological Science, 12*(2), 117-23

26 Toussaint, L. L., Owen, A. D., & Cheadle, A. (2011). Forgive to live: For-giveness, health, and longevity. *Journal of Behavioral Medicine, 35*(4), 375-386.

27 Seery, M. D., Holman, E. A., & Silver, R. C. (2010). Whatever does not kill us: Cumulative lifetime adversity, vulnerability, and resilience. *Journal of Personality and Social Psychology, 99*(6), 1025-1041.

28 Seery, M. D., Holman, E. A., & Silver, R. C. (2010). Whatever does not kill us: Cumulative lifetime adversity, vulnerability, and resilience. *Journal of Personality and Social Psychology, 99*(6), 1025-1041.

29 Seery, M. D., Holman, E. A., & Silver, R. C. (2010). Whatever does not kill us: Cumulative lifetime adversity, vulnerability, and resilience. *Journal of Personality and Social Psychology, 99*(6), 1025-1041.

30 Solomon, A. (2014) *How the worst moments in our lives make us who we are.* Speech presented at TedTalk, Vancouver.

31 Watson, D. L., & Tharp, R. G. (2013). *Self-directed behavior: Self-modification for personal adjustment* (10th ed.). Belmont, CA: Wadsworth Publishing.

32 Sheldon, K. M., & Lyubomirsky, S. (2006). Achieving sustainable gains in happiness: Change your actions, not your circumstances. *Journal of Happiness Studies, 7*(1), 55-86.

33 Lyubomirsky, S. (2008). *The how of happiness: A new approach to getting the life you want.* New York: Penguin Press, p40.

34 Diener, E., & Biswas-Diener, R. (2008). *Happiness: Unlocking the mysteries of psychological wealth.* Malden, MA: Blackwell Pub.

35 Wrzesniewski, A., McCauley, C., Rozin, P., & Schwartz, B. (1997). Jobs, ca-reers, and callings: People's relations to their work. *Journal of Research in Personality, 31*(1), 21-33.

36 Diener, E., & Biswas-Diener, R. (2008). *Happiness: Unlocking the mysteries of psychological wealth.* Malden, MA: Blackwell Pub.

37 Diener, E., & Biswas-Diener, R. (2008). *Happiness: Unlocking the mysteries of psychological wealth.* Malden, MA: Blackwell Pub.

38 Wrzesniewski, A., McCauley, C., Rozin, P., & Schwartz, B. (1997). Jobs, ca-reers, and callings: People's relations to their work. *Journal of Research in Personality, 31*(1), 93-135.

39 Cohen, S., Janicki-Deverts, D., Turner, R. B., & Doyle, W. J. (2014). Does hugging provide stress-buffering social support? A study of susceptibility to upper respiratory infection and illness. *Psychological Science, 26*(2), 135-147.

40   Brown, S. L., Nesse, R. M., Vinokur, A. D., & Smith, D. M. (2003). Providing social support may be more beneficial than receiving it: Results from a prospective study of mortality. *Psychological Science, 14*(4), 320-327.

41   Algoe, S. B., & Haidt, J. (2009). Witnessing excellence in action: The 'other-praising' emotions of elevation, gratitude, and admiration. *The Journal of Positive Psychology, 4*(2), 105-127.

42   King, L. A. (2001). The health benefits of writing about life goals. *Personality and Social Psychology Bulletin, 27*(7), 798-807.

43   Emmons, R. A. (2003). Personal goals, life meaning, and virtue: Wellsprings of a positive life. *Flourishing: Positive Psychology and the Life Well-lived,* 105-128.

44   Watson, D. L., & Tharp, R. G. (2013). *Self-directed behavior: Self-modification for personal adjustment* (10th ed.). Belmont, CA: Wadsworth Publishing.

45   Wilson, E. O. (1984). *Biophilia.* Cambridge, MA: Harvard University Press.

46   Capaldi, C. A., Dopko, R. L., & Zelenski, J. M. (2014). The relationship between nature connectedness and happiness: A meta-analysis. *Frontiers in Psychology, 5,* 976.

47   Howell, A. J., Dopko, R. L., Passmore, H., & Buro, K. (2011). Nature connectedness: Associations with well-being and mindfulness. *Personality and Individual Differences, 51*(2), 166-171.

48   Zelenski, J. M., & Nisbet, E. K. (2012). Happiness and feeling connected: The distinct role of nature relatedness. *Environment and Behavior, 46*(1), 3-23.

49   Ulrich, R. S., Simons, R. F., Losito, B. D., Fiorito, E., Miles, M. A., & Zelson, M. (1991). Stress recovery during exposure to natural and urban environments. *Journal of Environmental Psychology, 11*(3), 201-230.

50   Gray, T., & Birrell, C. (2014). Are biophilic-designed site office buildings linked to health benefits and high-performing occupants? *International Journal of Environmental Research and Public Health, 11*(12), 12204-12222.

51   Ulrich, R. (1984). View through a window may influence recovery from surgery. *Science, 224*(4647), 420-421.

52   Grinde, B., & Patil, G. G. (2009). Biophilia: Does visual contact with nature impact on health and well-being? *International Journal of Environmental Research and Public Health, 6*(9), 2332-2343.

53   Tennessen, C. M., & Cimprich, B. (1995). Views to nature: Effects on attention. *Journal of Environmental Psychology, 15*(1), 77-85.

54 Annerstedt, M., & Wahrborg, P. (2011). Nature-assisted therapy: Systematic review of controlled and observational studies. *Scandinavian Journal of Public Health, 39*(4), 371-388.

55 Lambert, G., Reid, C., Kaye, D., Jennings, G., & Esler, M. (2002). Effect of sunlight and season on serotonin turnover in the brain. *The Lancet, 360*(9348), 1840-1842.

56 Young, S. (2007). How to increase serotonin in the human brain without drugs. *Journal of Psychiatry and Neuroscience, 32*(6), 394-399.

57 The Nature Conservancy. (2011). *Connecting America's youth to nature* (Rep.). Retrieved http://www.nature.org/newsfeatures/kids-in-nature/youth-and-nature-poll-results.pdf

PART II

REVITALIZE

"To keep the body in good health is a duty...
otherwise we shall not be able to keep our mind strong and clear."

—Siddhartha Gautama

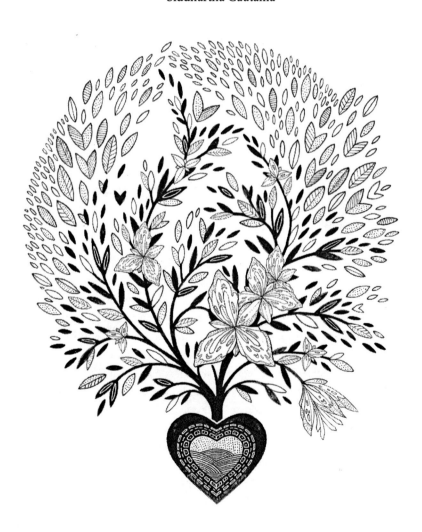

Chapter 5

Balance Your Body

Sustainability of the self, much like that for our world, is about maintenance and balance in order to achieve longevity. Although your biggest dreams in life may not have to do with your health, effective and thoughtful care for your mind, body, and environment can facilitate your path toward any grander goals you have. Indeed, being healthy holistically can help you not only to achieve longevity but also to think, act, socialize, and perform at your maximum potential on a daily basis.

While it is important to strengthen and maintain your inner well-being, it is equally important to strengthen and revitalize your body. In the next few chapters, you will learn what being holistically in shape entails and how to become more active with less effort, improve your postural health, and obtain quality, productive sleep.

A More Holistic Approach to Fitness

Being physically fit is not about being skinny, shedding a few pounds, or maintaining a body weight within a range suggested by fitness guidelines. One can be skinny but completely out of shape; one can shed a few pounds in ways detrimental to one's health; and one can maintain an ideal weight even when inactive for a whole month. It is not about what you look like or what measurements you have at one point in time, but about what you *do* on an ongoing basis.

While being in shape certainly can make your body look more toned as a natural consequence, being fit is actually functional. Because your mind and body are interconnected and affect one another, being physically fit can boost your mental health, decrease stress levels, make you happier, and improve your physical health, sleep quality, and energy levels.

Physical fitness is generally defined as the performance of the lungs, heart and muscles. Because your body is a complex system of many parts working together, building a strong, balanced body requires you to train in a way that considers *all* major components of physical fitness: body composition, flexibility, cardiorespiratory fitness, muscular endurance, and muscular strength. For example, if you run and lift weights regularly but lack flexibility, you would benefit from incorporating stretching into your workouts. Or, if you do only low-impact, restorative yoga, you would benefit from adding aerobic exercises to your routines. Instead of solely focusing on any part of your body or any one component of fitness, training your body holistically can help you better achieve overall body sustainability.

Don't Trust the Scale

Body composition, the first component of physical fitness, refers to the percentage of your body fat mass relative to your lean mass, including bones, organs, muscles, and ligaments. You can achieve a healthy body composition, minimizing fat mass, through balanced diets and exercise routines.

Since body weight is not all created equal, simply checking your weight on a scale does not truly indicate whether or not you are in good shape. For example, you will typically gain a few pounds after some strength-training exercises because muscle is denser than fat! This is a healthy increase in weight, as you will have increased your lean mass relative to your fat mass.

On the other hand, weight gain from excessive junk food consumption, which leads to an increase in your fat mass, indicates an unhealthy increase in your total body weight. If you wish to obtain more accurate information on your body composition, consult fitness trainers who have the proper measuring equipment. However, try to focus on what you do on an ongoing basis rather than on what specific measurements you have at any one point in time.

Stretching is Not Just for Gymnasts

The first image that comes to mind when I think about flexibility is gymnasts or acrobats doing crazy stunts. It is truly amazing how people can train their bodies to move in such a large range of motion! While most of us do not need to do 180-degree splits or backward bridges in our daily lives, stretching as a regular routine is still important to everyone and is not limited to dancers and performers.

Flexibility, the second component to physical fitness, refers to the ability of a specific joint or group of joints to move through an absolute range. Flexibility will not only let you move your joints freely through their full ranges of motions but will also help you prevent injuries, whether during athletic competitions or merely reaching for something from the top shelf at home. Flexibility also supports skeletal posture, prevents back pain, and increases blood circulation. Over the long term, it may even help maintain the elasticity of your arteries. A study found that flexibility is *independently* correlated with arterial stiffening (hardening of the arteries), an established risk factor for mortality and cardiovascular illnesses.[1]

Fortunately, stretching requires little time and can be done almost anywhere and anytime! For example, you can stretch in the morning to invigorate your body, before and after workouts to prevent injury, during your study or work breaks to stimulate blood flow after long hours of sitting, and at night to unwind before going to bed.

Note: To prevent injury, stretch only when the body is warmed up, because warming up increases blood flow and the temperature in your muscles, thus making them more elastic, like rubber bands. If you have been lying down or sitting for a while, make sure you move and walk around a little before diving into deep stretches.

On the following pages, you will find a few basic sample stretches for your larger muscle and joint groups guided by Los Angeles-based yoga instructor Krystal Huang. Remember to pay close attention to your body and take it slow, as everyone's level of flexibility is different. Moreover, keep in mind that flexibility involves many smaller components; for example, the flexibility of your calves is specific to just your calves and does not determine the flexibility of your right shoulder. So, being flexible overall requires you to practice stretching exercises that target multiple muscle and joint groups.

When you do these exercises, you should feel a stretch in your muscles, but once you feel pain, do not push yourself much further regardless of whether or not you have reached the completed pose.

Basic Sample Stretches

Figure 5-1. Cross-legged Seated Twist

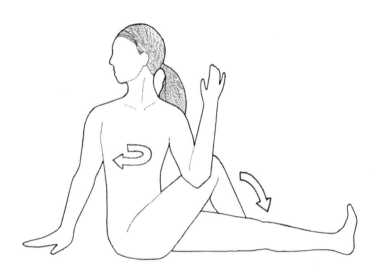

Benefits: Stretches hips and buttocks.

Set-up: Begin in a seated position with your legs extended straight in front of you. Bend and cross your right leg over your left leg so that your foot is planted by your left thigh. Keep your left leg straight.

Stretch: Place your right fingertips behind you, reach your left arm up, twist to your right, and place your arm over the outside of your right thigh. As you breathe, elongate through your spine on your inhales, and spin your ribs further into the twist on your exhales. Take 5 to 10 breaths. When you're ready, slowly come out of the pose and repeat on the other side.

Figure 5-2. Simple Forward Fold

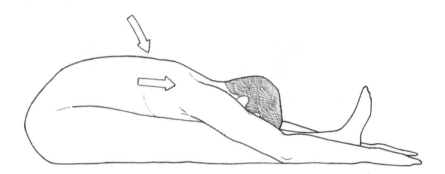

Benefits: Stretches all muscles on the backside of the body.

Set-up: Begin in a seated position with your legs extended straight in front of you.

Stretch: As you inhale, raise your arms and lift up and forward through your pelvis and the sides of the torso. Fold forward and place your hands by your ankles or feet. Keep your neck in line with your spine as you fold deeper into the pose by reaching forward with your torso and chest. Take 5-10 deep breaths and come out of the pose.

Figure 5-3. Low Cobra Pose

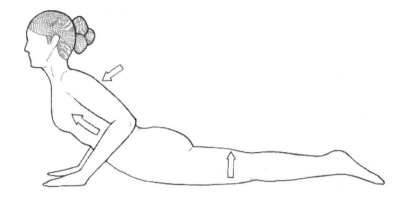

Benefits: Stretches the front of the body and strengthens the back extensors, thigh extensors, thigh internal rotators, shoulder extensors, and shoulder external rotators.

Set-up: Lie flat on your stomach. Bend your elbows and place your palms by your upper ribcage so that you form a 90-degree angle with your arms. (Make sure your elbows are stacked right over your wrists and not splaying out). Zip your legs together, and root down through your pubic bone and the tops of your feet.

Stretch: At your next inhale, lift your inner thighs and kneecaps, pull your hands back toward your heels, and lift your shoulders and sternum up and forward off the ground. Press your shoulder blades into your chest as you draw your navel into your spine. Draw your shoulders away from your ears, and lengthen all sides of the neck evenly. After a few more breaths, lower back down to the ground and rest.

Figure 5-4. Child's Pose

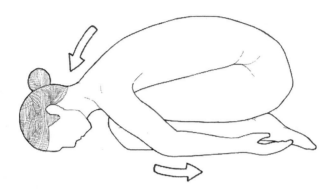

Benefits: Stretches the lower back, quadriceps and arms in an extended "Child's Pose."

Set-up: Begin in an upright kneeling position with your knees hip-width distance apart and big toes touching. Sit your hips back to your heels so that your shins, tops of feet, and all 10 toes are flat on the ground.

Stretch: Fold forward so your chest rests between your knees and your forehead touches the ground. Extend your arms back alongside your body or forward alongside your ears. Relax your inner groins, shoulders and head as your entire body sinks deeper into the ground.

Modification: For the Extended Child's Pose, reach your arms forward and plant your fingertips on the ground. Continue to sink your hips to your heels as you lengthen through the sides of your body and reach energetically forward through your arms and fingertips. Hold the pose for 10 breaths. When you're ready, relax your arms, and slowly rise back up to a seated position.

Figure 5-5. Upper Back Arm Stretch

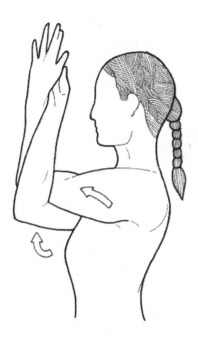

Benefits: Stretches triceps and releases tension in the upper back.

Set-up: Begin in a comfortable, cross-legged, seated position. Cross your right arm over your left arm at the elbows and wrists and place your palms together. Bring both of your elbows, wrists, and hands in line with your sternum as you keep your wrists and hands in front of your nose, aligned with the midline of your face.

Stretch: As you breathe in, widen your shoulder blades away from your spine. As you breathe out, stretch your arms farther up and away from your chest while you relax your shoulders away from your ears. Hold the pose for 10 breaths. When you're ready, uncross your arms, and repeat with your left arm crossed over your right arm.

Figure 5-6. Upper Back Arm Stretch II

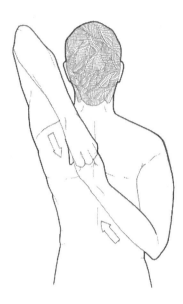

Benefits: Stretches triceps and upper back and opens the shoulders.

Set-up: Begin in a comfortable, cross-legged, seated position, and extend your arms out to a *T*.

Stretch: Reach your left arm down and back so that the back of your hand is flat against your upper back. Reach your right arm up and back so that your right hand meets your left hand. Clasp your fingertips, or hold a strap between your hands if your fingers cannot touch. As you breathe in and out, draw the bottom tip of your left shoulder blade toward your spine, and spread the bottom tip of your right shoulder blade away from your spine. Hold the pose for 10 breaths. When you're ready, release your arms, and repeat with your left arm on top.

Do Your Part to Train Your Heart

Why is it not accurate to judge how fit someone is by merely examining how toned he or she looks? Because, while looking lean might indicate that the person has balanced muscles, it does not reveal how healthy one's heart and lungs are.

Cardiorespiratory fitness (the third element to physical fitness) is so important for long-term physical health, because it indicates how well your heart and lungs are able to pump blood and deliver oxygen and other nutrients to the rest of your body.

Regardless of how toned your muscles are, you will benefit from having regular cardio exercises. In fact, the benefits of being lean may be limited to only people who are both lean *and* cardio-fit. Even after taking into account potentially confounding factors such as lifestyle, age, and health history, lean but unfit men were twice as likely to die from all causes than lean men who were cardio-fit.[2] Perhaps this drastic difference can be attributed to the overwhelming amount of benefits from cardio-fitness: lower risks for cardiovascular diseases or type 2 diabetes, lower blood pressure and cholesterol levels, healthier body composition, better sleep quality, decreased stress levels, etc.

Regular aerobic exercise is also one of the most effective ways to fight and delay the aging process. While brain volume (which reflects the brain's numerous functions) naturally decreases as we age, cardio exercises have been shown to slow down, and even reverse, this process in aging adults.[3-7] Because both your lungs and your heart are organs that impact the functioning of your entire body, keeping yourself cardio-fit is one of the most direct ways to keep your whole body healthy.

To gain the proven health benefits from cardio-training, Centers for Disease Control and Prevention (CDC) recommends the following amounts of aerobic exercises for adults per week (see Table 5-1).

Table 5-1. Recommended Amounts of Aerobic Exercises for Adults[8]

	Activity per Week
Option 1	2.5 hours of moderate-intensity aerobic activity
Option 2	1 hour and 15 minutes of high-intensity aerobic activity
Option 3	An equivalent mix of moderate- and high-intensity aerobic activities (where 2 minutes of moderate aerobic activity equals 1 minute of high-intensity aerobic activity)

Keep in mind that you do not need to do these activities all at once. If your schedule cannot afford you hours of continuous free time, just make sure that your exercises involve ongoing movements that speed up your heart rate at sustained levels for at least 10 minutes at a time. So, you can spread out your aerobic exercises into smaller chunks throughout your week. And, while these are admittedly minimum activity levels, you will obtain even greater health benefits if you exceed these recommended levels.

Examples of moderate-intensity aerobic activities include brisk walking, water aerobics, bike-riding with minimal incline levels, playing doubles tennis, rowing, etc. In moderately intense aerobic activities, you should feel your heart pumping harder and faster than usual but still be able to easily talk to your friends. Therefore, your dance courses, yoga sessions, Pilates classes, and crossfit workouts all count toward aerobic exercising if they keep your heart rate up for at least 10 minutes at a time.

High-intensity workout activities include jogging, running, swimming laps, bike-riding over hills or at high speed, basketball, etc. These exercises should get you breathing hard, making it difficult for you to talk to your friends without catching your breath.

Work Your Muscles to Prevent Trouble

Training your muscles, whether at home or at the gym, will address the final two elements of physical fitness: *muscular endurance* and *muscular strength*. Healthy muscles can help people—especially the elderly—to improve balance and decrease the risk of falling. They are also beneficial for overall bone health and maintaining good posture. Because you will lose your muscles if you don't use them, keeping your body toned requires you to work your muscles regularly.

Muscular endurance is the ability of your muscles to produce force repeatedly without tiring. For example, when you increase your number of repetitions for sit-ups from 20 to 25, you are training your muscles for endurance.

Muscular strength is the maximum amount of force a certain muscle can exert. If you begin by holding two pounds of weights this week while doing sit-ups, and then increase it to four pounds while doing sit-ups next week, you will be targeting abdominal muscular strength.

However, muscular endurance and muscular strength often go hand-in-hand, and can be trained simultaneously.

The CDC recommends muscle-strengthening activities involving all major muscle groups two or more days weekly.[9] These include working your legs, hips, back, abdomen, chest, shoulders, and arms. In order to obtain health benefits from strength training, your exercises should work your muscles to a point where you feel like it is becoming difficult to do another repetition of that movement. So, pay attention to how your muscles feel while you exercise. Are you getting that burning sensation from your muscles working, or does your activity feel effortless?

You can improve your muscular strength and endurance by lifting weights, performing resistance training, or taking workout classes that create that burning sensation in your muscles. You can also incorporate more muscle work into your daily routines, such as carrying grocery baskets, working strenuously in your garden, or walking up stairs instead of taking the elevator.

Chapter Summary

A More Holistic Approach to Fitness

Being in shape is more about what you do on an ongoing basis rather than how you look or how much you weigh at one point in time. Because your fitness level directly reflects your health, making a conscious effort to train your body in a balanced manner can help you perform at your maximum potential in the short run and achieve longevity in the long term.

Don't Trust the Scale

A desirable **body composition** minimizes fat mass relative to the rest of the body mass. The key to a healthy body composition involves eating a balanced diet and planning balanced exercises.

Stretching is Not Just for Gymnasts

Flexibility can improve overall health and decrease risks of injury. Make sure to warm up prior to stretching, and deepen your stretches slowly to prevent pulling muscles in the process.

Do Your Part and Train Your Heart

Cardio fitness is extremely important for long-term health, as it indicates how healthy and strong your heart and lungs are. Incorporate regular aerobic exercises that speed up your heart rate at sustained levels into your weekly routines!

Work Your Muscles to Prevent Trouble

Improving **muscular strength** and **endurance** can help to improve your balance, decrease the risk of falling, improve your postural health, and prevent you from being easily fatigued by physical activity. Take every chance you can get to put your muscles to work!

Chapter 6

Gain With No Pain

The human body is made to *move*. Think about it: We used to trek over vast areas of land just to collect food in the wild. Now, many of us spend the majority of our time sitting around. When we are active, we improve our blood circulation and enable the nutrients and oxygen we take in to efficiently reach and nourish all parts of our bodies. However, when we remain inactive for prolonged periods of time, our bodies cannot function at their maximum potentials.

In fact, inactivity is a key risk factor for noncommunicable diseases such as cancer, diabetes, and cardiovascular disease. According to the World Health Organization, around 3.2 million deaths each year can be attributed to insufficient physical activity.[10] Moreover, while the amount of calories we consume on average has increased since the 1980s, the amount of energy we expend on average has decreased. This has led to imbalances that very likely contribute to the ongoing rise in obesity rates.[11]

Now that many of our modern sedentary routines have deviated from the active lifestyles our bodies are adapted to, we must make conscious effort to engage in more movement and physical activity.

Get Fit with Activities that Fit *You*

As discussed in Chapter 2 (see "Find Stress Reducers that Fit *You*"), the key to incorporating new activities into your established routines is to find the types of activities that suit your interests and lifestyle. To successfully become more active, then, you can begin by asking yourself these questions:

- **Current lifestyle:** How active are you already? Does your work life revolve around physical activity (professional marathon-running, farming, running errands, etc.), or does it revolve around tasks you do at a desk or at home?

- **Activity type:** What types of physical activities interest you? What activities does your health status allow? Do you prefer activities that are more leisurely, or more competitive? Low impact, or high intensity? By yourself, or with a group? Which fitness components do you need to dedicate more time to?

- **Frequency and duration**: What types of activities can you incorporate into your schedule? How often can you do them? Do you have short breaks scattered throughout your day? Or do you have hours of free time at once?

- **Location**: According to your lifestyle and local environment, where can you engage in more physical activity? At home, or at a local gym? Indoors, or outdoors? How "walkable" is your city? Can you walk or bike instead of driving or taking public transportation?

Using your answers to these questions, think about what types of activities you can most easily incorporate into your lifestyle to efficiently and effectively become more active.

Work With Your Body

No matter what types of activities you plan, it is important to pay attention to how your body responds to training so you can avoid injuries and prevent overworking your body. We will consider how you can plan safe workouts according to the following principles of exercise training:

- **Progression**: Increase the duration and intensity of your workouts slowly, and work your way up to your goal. Also, make sure to warm up before exercising. For example, you can walk briskly or jog for five minutes before beginning a more intensive workout.

- **Recuperation**: Listen to your body. Especially after higher-intensity workouts or weight-training, give your body time to heal.

- **Reversibility**: Fitness is reversible. If you ran a marathon five years ago but have not run at all since then, you will have lost that level of fitness and will have to progressively rework your way up again.

- **Overload**: If you want to increase your muscle strength, you will have to start lifting heavier weights than what you were lifting before. If you want to increase your running endurance, you will have to run for a longer duration of time than you did the last time you trained. In other words, to become fitter than you were before or are now, you will have to push yourself a little past your current limits.

- **Specificity**: *Specificity* refers to how the effects of exercises are limited to what they are used for. For example, building arm muscles will not increase your leg muscles, and stretching will not necessarily increase your cardiorespiratory endurance. So make sure you incorporate a variety of exercises into your routine to engage your entire body in a more holistic manner.[12]

Don't Take the Short Cut

I used to complain that I was too busy to go to the gym to work out. However, Michael Merbaum, PhD, Professor of Behavioral Psychology at Washington University in St. Louis, challenged me to think about exercise in a new light. Instead of trying to block out hours at a time to engage in some sort of physical exercise, Dr. Merbaum suggested that busy people can become more active by simply building mini-exercises into their established routines. Here are some examples:

- Get more aerobic exercise by walking at a brisk pace or biking to your destination instead of driving. This will also decrease your personal ecological footprint.

- If you were already planning on walking somewhere, leave an extra 10 minutes early and take a longer route to your destination to increase your walking distance.

- If you are already holding some shopping bags, grocery baskets, or something heavy, do a few arm exercises while holding them.

- If you are already standing, flex your calves, thighs, and butt muscles; dance around the space you are in; do some squats if possible; or perform some feet rocks (see the section in Chapter 7 called, "A Little Work Will Go a Long Way").

- Work your leg and butt muscles by walking up stairs instead of taking the elevator. If you live on a high floor, walk up a few flights of stairs first, then switch to the elevator.

- If your work life requires you to sit for hours at a time, do some leg and butt flexes at the desk, tap your feet once in a while, and take regular stretch-breaks. Or, if possible, obtain a height-adjustable desk so you can alternate between standing up and sitting down.

Notice how none of these mini-workouts require you to change into active wear, get sweaty and shower afterward, or block out hours of free time at once. You simply need to get creative with your current routine and seize every opportunity to move around more, increase your walking distance, and work your muscles more than you already do.

As mentioned previously, inactivity for prolonged periods of time contributes to poor blood flow within your body. This may then lead to blood clots forming in your leg veins, a condition known as *deep vein thrombosis*.[13] More alarming is that, if these clots break off and travel through your body, you may develop *pulmonary embolism* (blockage of one of the pulmonary arteries), which can be life-threatening! Thankfully, though, you can easily prevent poor blood circulation by simply becoming more active.

No matter how sedentary your lifestyle, just make sure you are never in one position for too long (apart from lying down to go to sleep). If you have an urge to move after sitting or standing in the same place for a while, that's your body's way of telling you that you need to move!

Chapter Summary

Get Fit with Activities that Fit You

To successfully adopt a more active lifestyle, find physical activities that are most suited for you. Think about how active you already are, what activities you are interested in, what condition your body is in, what components of fitness you need to spend more time on, what types of exercise your lifestyle permits, etc. Then, use your answers to these questions to see how you can best incorporate more physical activity into your current routine.

Work With Your Body

To prevent injury and to train your body efficiently, keep these exercise principles in mind: **progression, recuperation, reversibility, overload,** and **specificity.** Warm up before intensive workouts. Work your way up slowly in your exercises. Listen to your body constantly. Give it time to heal afterward. And, plan various exercises that target the different components of fitness, as well as different muscle groups within your body. By understanding how to safely, efficiently, and effectively strengthen your body, you will more easily achieve holistic physical fitness.

Don't Take the Short Cut

Becoming more active does not require you to get a gym membership. Instead, you can begin by looking to incorporate more movement into your existing lifestyle. When possible, walk longer distances, take the stairs instead of the elevator, take frequent stretch-breaks from sitting at your desk, obtain a standing desk for work, flex and engage your muscles when forced to sit or stand still for a long time, choose to carry something instead of using a cart, and so on. Whenever you get the chance—move!

Chapter 7

Mind Your Body

Check your posture. Are you sitting or standing upright? As I write this in a café, I cannot help noticing that more than half of the people around me are slouching. Did you know that bad posture can strain or pull your back or neck muscles and cause pain? Consider your posture from an architectural standpoint. For a building to last for a long time, it must have well-supported, well-balanced structures so that the building will not exert too much pressure on any particular side. Similarly, good posture will help you to maintain your skeletal health and prevent your spine from deteriorating.

As easy as it may be to simply tell yourself to sit up straight or stand up tall, adopting a healthy posture as an effortless habit is no simple task. The rest of this chapter will show you why correcting bad posture is so important, how you can strengthen your mind-body awareness, what a healthy posture involves, and which exercises you can do to improve your postural health.

I Have a Hunch That You Won't Want a Hunch

Slouching not only strains the neck and spine but also decreases one's lung capacity and ability to breathe out air.[14] For your entire body to function properly, however, it is extremely important for you to breathe smoothly so you can efficiently bring oxygen into your body and expel carbon dioxide. Julifer Day, a Los Angeles-based fitness trainer and the creator of "Day by Day Training," even commented that poor posture is like forcing your body to function with a chest cold—all the time!

Plus, sitting or standing upright can make you not only look more confident, but also *feel* more confident! A psychology study suggested that merely sitting upright in the face of stress can help maintain self-confidence, reduce negative mood and fear, and increase positive mood.[15] Who knew posture could have such a large impact over one's overall mental and physical health?

Check Yourself Out

The first step to improving posture is to tune in to your bodily positions, for example: becoming aware of your strides when you walk, of how your body moves when you bend down to pick something off the ground, of how your posture transitions from standing to sitting, etc. After all, if you are not aware of your posture and movements, how can you begin to improve them? (See also the "Take Control" section in Chapter 3.)

A great way to strengthen your mind-body connection is to set up frequent self-reminders to check in on your posture. For example, if you check your phone periodically, put a small sticker on its corner so that every time you see the sticker, you will be reminded to check and correct your posture. You can also set vibrating alarm clocks on your phone to go off every hour or at random times throughout your day. Every time it goes off, check your posture and correct it as necessary.

The key to setting up effective mind-body awareness cues is to find ones that are readily and frequently available and meaningful to you. After getting used to regularly checking your posture with the help of external reminders, you will soon find yourself naturally more attentive to your body's positions.

Body Architecture 101

Once you become more aware of your body's stance, you will have to know how to fix poor posture when it occurs. What does a healthy posture look like? This section contains tips to help you maintain the three healthy curvatures in your spine (Figure 7-1) while you sit, stand and sleep.[16] If you can, test out the tips as you read along so you know what having a good posture feels like and can correct yourself without external guides in the future.

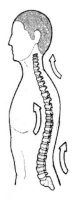

Figure 7-1. The Three Natural Curvatures in a Healthy Spine

1. A forward curve at the neck
2. A backward curve at the upper back
3. A forward curve at the lower back

Tips for Sitting Properly

- Keep your feet flat on the floor. Use a footrest if needed.

- Avoid crossing your legs; that increases blood pressure. Keep your ankles in front of your knees.

- Your knees should be at or below your hip level.

- Use a back support for your lower and middle back.

- Maintain the three natural curves in your back.

Regardless of how good a sitting posture you have, sitting for prolonged periods of time can still strain your body. Remember: Our bodies are made to move! So, set reminders to stand up every half-hour to stretch and walk around. Or, as fitness trainer Julifer Day suggests, periodically squeeze your butt while seated to reinforce that mind-body awareness link.

Tips for Standing Upright

- Wear two-strapped backpacks that distribute the weight evenly on both sides of your body, as opposed to one-sided bags that make you lean more in one direction. If you do carry one-sided bags, alternate the side you carry them on.

- Minimize the amount of time you wear high heels or uncomfortable shoes, as wearing them exerts stress on your body and forces you to arch your back in unnatural ways.

- Balance your weight equally between your feet.

- Soften your knees, and avoid locking them straight.

- Stand upright and tall, pulling your shoulders slightly backward.

- Engage your core muscles.

- Keep your head positioned directly in line with your shoulders, rather than backward, forward, or to one side.

Just as you are not meant to sit still for hours at once, standing still for too long can also strain your body. If you are forced to stand in one place for a while, move around as much as you can within that space, shifting your weight back and forth between your heels and your toes, or between one foot and the other foot.

Tips for Sleeping Correctly

- Get a mattress or topper you feel comfortable sleeping on.

- Test out and use a pillow that supports your sleeping posture.

- Sleep on your side or your back instead of your stomach.

- If you sleep on your side, place a pillow between your legs to prevent your bones from exerting pressure on one another.

- If you sleep on your back, place a pillow under your knees to support the natural arches in your back.

Correcting poor posture will require constant alterations of your ongoing movements and stances. After all, just as you breathe whether you are conscious of it or not, you hold a posture no matter where you are or what you are doing. Thus, even though improving postural health for the long run may take a few weeks of mental focus and regular mind-and-body engagement, the beneficial effects of having a good posture as a natural habit can follow you for a lifetime.

A Little Work Will Go a Long Way

Because your body is one whole system of many smaller parts working together, living a holistically healthy lifestyle can help to improve your postural health. Thus, take care of your inner well-being; stretch regularly; keep your muscles fit; stay active; sleep well; eat a balanced diet; and stay hydrated.

Other than when you are lying down fully relaxed and preparing to sleep, every other position, including sitting, requires you to engage some of your muscles. Therefore, you may even feel your back and core muscles burning when you begin to adopt a healthier posture, especially if you do not have strong core and back muscles or a flexible back, chest, hips, and shoulders. However, do not give up—I promise that maintaining healthy postures will get easier over time.

On the following pages, Morgana Mellet, a New York-based personal trainer, Pilates and yoga instructor, and founder of MOMO Momentum Training w/ Morgana LLC (www.momotraining.life), shares with us a set of simple exercises you can do daily to encourage healthy postures in your whole body. With minimal time and equipment needed, you will be able to practice these exercises regularly at your gym, or even just in the comforts of your own home.

Working Toward Healthy Postures

Equipment:
1. Mat
2. Chair
3. Countertop to hold onto
4. Yoga strap or belt (optional)
5. Yoga block (optional)

Attire: Comfortable clothing that you can move in. All exercises are intended to be performed barefoot.

Figure 7-1. Relaxation Pose

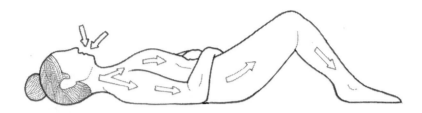

Benefits: By placing the spine and pelvis in a relaxed, neutral position and allowing your breathing to deepen, you encourage your body to relax and release patterns of tension and poor posture. The relaxation pose cleans the slate to prepare you to develop postural awareness.

Set-up: Rest on a mat facing up with your knees bent, feet on the mat (parallel and hip-width distance apart), and arms resting comfortably by your side.

Movement: Allow your eyes to become heavy and/or closed. Focus on your breathing moving slowly in and out of your body. Scan your body for places of tension or discomfort. Send your breathing into these areas, exhaling the tension out of your body.

Modifications: If your knees tend to collapse inwards, place a yoga block between your thighs to keep them parallel and hip-width distance apart. Rest your hands comfortably on your chest or abdomen if preferred.

Repetitions: Remain in the pose for at least 1 minute, and try to work toward holding the pose for 5 to 10 minutes.

Figure 7-2. Neck Strengthener

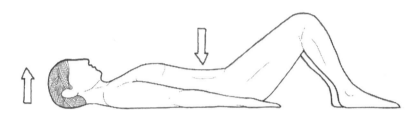

Benefits: This exercise strengthens the muscles of the neck and addresses your tendency to stick the chin forward when you are texting, eating, washing dishes, or engaged in other daily activities.

Set-up: Rest on the mat facing up with your knees bent, feet on the mat (parallel and hip-width distance apart), and arms comfortably by your side.

Movement: Press the back of your head into the floor slightly, tucking in your chin. Feel the muscles in the front of your neck engage. Keeping your chin slightly tucked, lift your head off the floor *only enough to slip a piece of paper under the back of your head*. Do not try to lift your head high; the goal is for your head to barely hover above the floor.

Repetitions: 10 repetitions for 5 seconds each. Gradually build up to 10 seconds.

Figure 7-3. Abdominals/Plank Pose

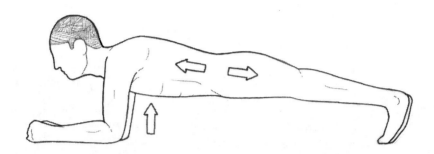

Benefits: This exercise strengthens and engages the deepest abdominal muscles for improved postural and lower back support.

Set-up: Lie on the floor facing down, propped up on your forearms.

Movement: Tuck your toes, pull your bellybutton into your spine, and keep it engaged throughout the exercise. Press into your forearms, and lift your body off the floor into a straight plank position. Engage the muscles of your core, thighs, and glutes, and press into your forearms. Check that your hips are in line with your head and have not gone upward or sagged toward the floor.

Modifications: To make this position less challenging, keep your knees on the ground.

Repetitions: Hold the plank position for 10 seconds, rest, and repeat 6 times. Eventually build up to holding the plank position for a full minute.

Figure 7-4. Glute Bridges

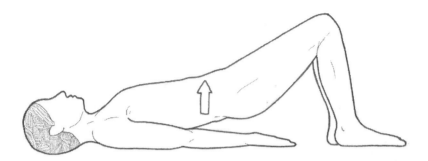

Benefits: This exercise strengthens the muscles in the back of your hips and thighs that support standing, walking, and other physical activities.

Set-up: Rest on the floor facing up with your knees bent, feet on the floor (parallel and hip-width distance apart), arms by your side, and palms pressed gently into the floor.

Movement: Pull your bellybutton in, and press your lower back into the mat. Engage your buttocks and inner thighs. Lift your hips a few inches off the floor, continuing to engage the muscles of the glutes, hamstrings, inner thighs, and abdominals. *Do not* raise your hips all the way up; if you do, you will not engage the targeted muscles. Roll down through the spine, lengthening out the lower back until you return to a relaxed spine position.

Modifications: Place a block between your thighs to keep your feet and legs parallel and hip-width distance apart.

Repetitions: Repeat 10 times, holding for 5 seconds at the top, and rolling slowly and smoothly through the spine to go up and down.

Figure 7-5. Back

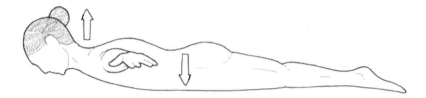

Benefits: This exercise strengthens the upper back and reverses the forward rounding posture common in everyday activities.

Set-up: Lie on your chest, bring your legs together, and extend your arms out to the side with your palms facing down.

Movement: Pull your bellybutton up and into your spine, and keep it there to protect your lower back. Press your hands into the floor, and lift your face, neck, and upper back slightly off the floor. Lift your hands off the floor. Focus on engaging your upper-middle back and keeping the abdominals engaged. Keep your chin tucked so your neck is in line with your spine.

Modifications: If this bothers your lower back, try pulling your bellybutton in more deeply and opening your legs slightly apart.

Repetitions: Hold this position for 4 seconds. Repeat 10 times.

Figure 7-6. Shoulders

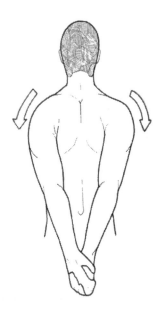

Benefits: This exercise strengthens the muscles of the upper back and opens the chest, reverses the forward rounding posture common to everyday activities, and opens the front of the shoulders and chest.

Set-up: Stand or sit with feet slightly wider than hip-width distance apart, and clasp your hands behind your back.

Movement: Roll your shoulders up and back. Press your shoulder-blades together and down your back until you feel the front of your chest opening.

Modifications: Join your palms together if you can. If your shoulders are tight and this is not possible, interlace your fingers, or use a yoga strap.

Repetitions: Hold the position for 10 seconds. Repeat 5 times or throughout the day.

Figure 7-7. Squats

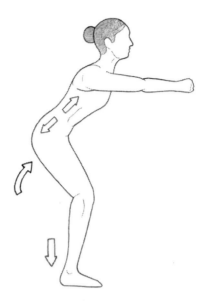

Benefits: This exercise strengthens the muscles responsible for healthy sitting and standing postures.

Set-up: Sit on a chair with your hips, knees, and feet flexed at a 90-degree angle. Be sure you can comfortably sit with your feet planted on the floor. Your feet should be parallel and hip-width distance apart.

Movement: Lean forward by folding at the hips. Look ahead and slightly upwards, keeping your spine flat. Pull your bellybutton into your spine, and press your feet into the ground to come up into a standing position. Go through the same movements in reverse to sit back down on the chair. Make sure your knees are tracking over your toes and you are pressing into your feet, engaging the thighs, glutes, and abdominals, and maintaining a straight, neutral spine.

Modifications: If the movement is difficult, reach your arms forward, or use a solid object (e.g., a countertop) to facilitate the movement.

Repetitions: Repeat slowly for 10 times, and mindfully go through these same motions any time you sit down or stand up from the seated position.

Figure 7-8. Feet Rocks

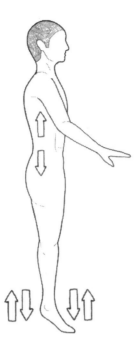

Benefits: This exercise strengthens your feet and ankles and facilitates healthier postural alignment.

Set-up: Stand with your feet parallel and hip-width distance apart, and hold on-to a countertop.

Movement: Pull your bellybutton into your spine, open up your chest, and gently engage your upper-middle back. Check to see that your neck is in line with your spine and that your gaze is directly forward. Rock back and forth, shifting your weight backward onto your heels with your toes lifted, then forward onto the balls of your feet with your heels lifted.

Modifications: Make the rocking motion smaller or bigger, depending on what feels more comfortable to you.

Repetitions: Repeat 10 times, back and forth.

Chapter Summary

I Have a Hunch That You Won't Want a Hunch

Poor posture can contribute to poor breathing, back or neck pain, stress, negative moods, lowered self-esteem, feelings of isolation, and deterioration of your skeletal health over time. Its negative impacts on both mental and physical health underscore the importance of adopting better posture as a long-lasting, natural habit.

Check Yourself Out

The first step to adopting healthier postures is to become **aware** of your bodily positions. Set frequent reminders to check in on your posture to strengthen your mind-body connection.

Body Architecture 101

Once you become aware of your posture, you will need to know how to correct it. Whether you are sitting, standing, or sleeping, try to maintain the three natural curves in your back as often as you can for a healthier spine. Regardless of how healthy your posture is, however, remember that staying in any position for too long can strain your body. So don't forget to move every so often.

A Little Work Will Go a Long Way

Maintaining healthy posture may be a challenge, but it is one that is definitely worth overcoming. In addition to living a holistically healthy lifestyle, try to incorporate some exercises that target postural health to facilitate this process. Over time, your body will adjust, and maintaining good postures will become a natural habit.

Chapter 8

Sleep Productively

We all sleep within our daily routines at different times, durations, and frequencies. But why do we need to ensure that we sleep well, enough, and at the right hours?

The truth is, sleeping is far from being unproductive—it serves numerous functions beyond reducing fatigue. While you cannot actively do anything after you fall asleep, your body continues to repair and revitalize itself so that you will be able to function at your peak potential mentally and physically during your waking hours.[17]

Sleep Your Way to Better Health

Most of us know the effects of sleep deprivation: We feel sleepy, sometimes moody, and are unable to concentrate the next day. However, the negative impacts extend well beyond just making us want to lie down and take a nap.

Here are just some of the immediate and long-term effects of inadequate sleep:

- Sleep deprivation can throw your body's hunger and fullness cues out of whack and make you more likely to overeat.[18] (See the "Master Your Body's Language" section in Chapter 9.)
- The detrimental effects of even moderate sleep loss can be seen through the sudden increase in heart attacks and car accidents the day after springtime daylight savings, when everyone loses just one hour of sleep.[19-21]
- Cognitive impairment from over 17 hours of wakefulness has been compared to having a blood alcohol concentration of 0.05%, a level considered to be legal alcohol intoxication in many Western industrialized countries![22]
- Lack of sleep has been linked to many chronic diseases such as cardiovascular disease, obesity, depression, and diabetes.[23-26]

As you can see, getting the right amount of sleep is an integral part of a healthy lifestyle.

The National Sleep Foundation recommends seven to nine hours of sleep for adults aged 18–64 and seven to eight hours for adults aged 65 and older.[27] However, because everyone's bodies are different and everyone's ideal sleep duration changes with age, the best way to find out the exact amount of sleep you need is to listen to your body. If you regularly go to sleep at 11 p.m. and wake up naturally at 5 a.m. every morning, six hours may work fine for your body. However, if you go to sleep at 11 p.m. every night and are groggily woken up by your 5 a.m. alarm clock every morning, your body probably needs more sleep for it to function optimally.

If you have no idea how much sleep is ideal for you, you can keep a sleep log to better understand your body's sleep requirements. In your sleep log, keep track of your sleep and wake times, sleep duration, how easily you fall asleep, how you feel when you wake up, etc. You can also find applications or sleep-tracking guidelines online that can guide you through this journaling process. After a few weeks, you can then analyze your report to see what duration of sleep best suits your lifestyle but still enables you to wake up feeling invigorated.

The better you sleep at night, the less likely you will feel an afternoon slump after lunchtime. However, if you still often feel the need to nap during the day, you should plan ahead and incorporate regular naps into your schedule. In a study on overcoming afternoon sleepiness, researchers found that naps trumped both using caffeine and getting more nighttime sleep in effectiveness.[28] Plus, you don't need to dedicate much time for napping for it to be effective.

Surprisingly, 10-minute afternoon naps were found to be the most recuperative compared to 5-minute, 20-minute and 30-minute naps.[29] While 30 minutes of napping resulted in a period of impaired alertness and performance in the nappers right after waking, 10 minutes of napping had no such side effects and produced only immediate benefits.[30] So, if you can recharge your mind and body by sparing 10 to 30 minutes of your afternoon time, why not give it a try? To make your naps as effective as possible, make them a regular part of your routine, and find some place cool, dark and quiet for them.

No matter what sleep schedule or napping habits you have, the key to healthier sleep patterns is to become more attentive to your body. Instead of constantly fighting against your body's signs of fatigue or overly relying on external substances to keep you feeling energized, remember that fatigue is your body's way of telling you that it is not functioning optimally and you need to change your lifestyle habits to help it recuperate. If you have no underlying illness and already have a healthy mind, a balanced diet, and an engagement in regular physical activity, any signs of fatigue probably stem from lack of sleep. If this is the case for you, focus on incorporating catnaps into your routine, sleeping a little more, or going to bed a little earlier so your body can properly restore itself from the inside out.

Bedtimes are Not Just for Kids

Not only is your sleep duration within a day important, so is *when* you go to bed. Our bodies operate on *circadian rhythms*—which depend partly on genetics and partly on environmental factors (daylight, ambient temperature, etc.) to regulate sleep, energy levels, and appetite. Therefore, we all have ideal bedtimes that work best for each of our bodies.

During our nighttime sleep, our bodies cycle chronologically through the following stages of sleep every 90 to 110 minutes:

Non-Rapid Eye Movement (NREM) Sleep
Stage 1: Light sleep, in-between being awake and being asleep.
Stage 2: Body temperature drops; becoming disengaged from surroundings.
Stages 3 & 4 (deep sleep): Most restorative sleep—blood pressure drops, breathing rate slows, muscles relax, blood supply to muscles increases, tissue growth and repair occur, energy is restored, hormones are released (important for growth and development).

Rapid-Eye Movement (REM) Sleep
Brain is active, and dreaming begins—eyes move rapidly, muscles are turned off, brain regions used in learning are stimulated.

Although the exact functions of deep sleep and REM sleep are still not perfectly understood, what is known is that the amount of time we spend within each stage of sleep changes as the night progresses. During the first sleep cycles earlier in the night, we enter deep sleep for relatively longer periods of time and REM sleep for shorter periods.[31] Later into the night, deep sleep durations decrease, and REM sleep durations increase.[32] By early morning, people spend most of their sleep times within stages 1, 2, and REM sleep, and not as much time in deep sleep. Due to the important functions of both deep sleep and REM sleep, going to bed early and getting the right amount of sleep allows your body to restore itself overnight most effectively.

Matt Walker, PhD, head of the Sleep and Neuroimaging Lab at the University of California, Berkeley, suggested that the best time to go to bed (to ensure sufficient amounts of both deep sleep and REM sleep) is sometime between 8 p.m. and 12 a.m.[33] However, note that every person's ideal bedtime within this "early" range is different. Some people are born to be early birds; others, to be night owls. While sleeping guidelines are helpful as references, you still need to get in touch with your body and experiment, using your sleep log, to find out what sleep routine works best for you and your lifestyle.

While regular sleep schedules are ideal, sometimes they are just not possible for people working night shifts or having that occasional night out. If this is your situation, you can still improve your sleep quality by obtaining blackout shades so you will not be woken up when daylight creeps into your bedroom. For optimum health, however, get to know what ranges of duration and bedtime work best for your body, and try to set regular sleep schedules, taking this information into account.

The Proper Presleep Prep

With today's abundance of artificial lighting and controlled indoor room temperatures, many of us don't feel naturally sleepy when we are supposed to. For example, blue lights from backlit screens, or bluish-white light bulbs (which mimic the color temperature of morning daylight) have been shown to suppress melatonin production, making it harder for people to fall asleep.[34] In addition, a recent study on some preindustrial societies that still exist and live in Tanzania, Namibia, and Bolivia and are unaffected by artificial lighting revealed that the onset of sleep is linked to the *natural drop in ambient temperature*—which most of us do not feel anymore, due to artificial thermostats.[35]

To promote better sleep quality at night, then, you can simulate the natural outdoor environmental changes in your own home. For example, avoid using electronic devices with backlit screens right before you sleep, and adjust your indoor lights to mimic natural lighting, which transitions from white light into yellow light and then fades out slowly as you near your bedtime. Conveniently, dimming your lights in the evenings can also decrease your electricity use, thus lowering your utility bills and your environmental impact.

To mimic the natural drop in outdoor temperature, open the window, turn on your fan, turn down your heater, wear less clothing at night, or use thinner blankets when you sleep. Instead of maintaining the "perfect" indoor room temperature the whole day, let it fluctuate as it naturally does outdoors: warmer in daytime, cooler after sunset.

Other ways to promote better sleep include: getting in enough physical activity during the day, and avoiding sleep right after drinking caffeinated beverages, smoking cigarettes, drinking alcohol, or eating a big meal. Caffeine and nicotine will keep you awake at night, while alcohol, despite being a sedative, will disrupt your normal sleeping cycles and prevent you from entering deep sleep, the most important stage for repairing and reenergizing your body. Meanwhile, going to bed with a full stomach may cause acid reflux, which can make you feel uncomfortable and keep you awake, as well as damage your insides. So, try to give yourself at least two hours to digest or process your food, caffeine, nicotine, and alcohol before you go to sleep.

If you ever find yourself waking up in the middle of the night after a few hours of sleep, don't panic and don't reach for your sleeping pills right away. Historian Roger Ekirch discovered from documents and literature from preindustrial European times that people used to have several chunks of sleep at night (called *polyphasic sleep*),[36] which is also how many animals sleep in the wild. Additional research also suggested that *biphasic sleep* (two chunks of sleep) may naturally occur when people are not influenced by sleep distractions at night (e.g., listening to music) or artificial lighting after sunset (which results in shorter light hours).[37] These findings raise the idea that middle-of-the-night insomnia, one of the most commonly reported forms of insomnia, may not necessarily be a problem but might, in fact, be normal. So, next time you wake up in the middle of the night, don't fret; unless you suspect that you might have underlying health or lifestyle problems that cause you to wake up in the middle of the night, just lie peacefully in bed, meditate or pray, or get up and do something (in dim lighting) until you are sleepy again.

If you have a hard time falling asleep to begin with, however, try these tips to put you in the mood to sleep:

- Scent your sleeping space with natural lavender.

- Listen to calming music.

- Envision a relaxing scene (the beach, a waterfall, etc.).

- Take a warm shower or bath before going to sleep.

- Drink relaxing herbal teas, such as chamomile tea.

- Soak your hands and feet in warm water before sleeping, or wear socks to sleep.

- Try *progressive relaxation*: lie down and focus on relaxing each part of your body for three seconds each—from your feet to your calves, knees, thighs, rear, abdomen, chest, shoulders, arms, hands, fingers, neck, jaw, face, and eyes—while maintaining slow, rhythmic breathing.

Last but not least, try relaxing breathing exercises that can gradually slow down your breathing and heart-rate. In the following section, New York-based yoga instructor Nicole Bell shares with us a simple conscious-breathing exercise you can practice nightly before going to bed to help you snooze away more easily.

Breathe Your Way to Sleep

Set-up: Lie down on your bed facing up and find a resting place for your head, neck, and spine. Rest one hand on your chest and the other on your belly.

Mind–body awareness: Become conscious of your breathing. As you inhale, feel your chest and abdomen rise with your hands. As you exhale, feel your chest and abdomen slowly fall as you release your breath into the air around you.

Conscious breathing: Through your nose, inhale for three counts, then exhale for three counts. Continue to focus on your breathing as you inhale and exhale.

Slowing down: When you feel settled, deepen your breathing. Slowly increase your inhale and exhale counts. Elongate your breathing by exhaling for twice as long as you inhale (e.g., inhale 5 counts, exhale 10 counts). This will naturally slow your breathing, putting you into a more relaxed state.

Dozing off: Continue focusing on your deep breaths. Allow your eyelids to fall closed during this breathing exercise, and breathe your way to sleep...

Chapter Summary

Sleep Your Way to Better Health

Sleep is far from being unproductive; it allows your body to repair and recover so that you will be able to perform at your peak potential mentally and physically during your waking hours. So, prioritize sleep and listen to your body to find out your personal and ideal duration of sleep. If you plan on taking afternoon naps, keep them short (as little as 10 minutes) and regular, and nap in dark, cool places.

Bedtimes are Not Just for Kids

Going to sleep early (according to your body's biological clock) can help ensure that you get sufficient amounts of both deep sleep and REM sleep overnight, thus allowing your body to most effectively restore itself. While experts suggest sleeping between 8 p.m. and 12 a.m., you will have to find your own ideal bedtime through personal experience or the use of sleep logs.

The Proper Presleep Prep

The better you sleep at night, the more productive your body will be while you sleep, and the more revitalized you will feel in the morning. Get yourself in the mood to sleep by making the proper presleep preparations: dim your lights as you near your bedtime; set up a cooler environment to sleep in; give your body a few hours to digest your dinner and process your alcohol, nicotine, and caffeine before going to bed; and do some stress-relief and relaxation activities before your bedtime.

Part References

1   Yamamoto, K., Kawano, H., Gando, Y., Iemitsu, M., Murakami, H., Sanada, K., . . . Miyachi, M. (2009). Poor trunk flexibility is associated with arterial stiffening. *American Journal of Physiology: Heart and Circulatory Physiology, 297*(4).

2   Lee, C. D., Blair, S. N., & Jackson, A. S. (1999). Cardiorespiratory fitness, body composition, and all-cause and cardiovascular disease mortality in men. *American Society for Clinical Nutrition, 69*(3), 373-380.

3   Burzynska, A. Z., Chaddock-Heyman, L., Voss, M. W., Wong, C. N., Gothe, N. P., Olson, E. A., . . . Kramer, A. F. (2014). Physical activity and cardiorespiratory fitness are beneficial for white matter in low-fit older adults. *PLoS ONE, 9*(9).

4   Colcombe, S. J., Erickson, K. I., Scalf, P. E., Kim, J. S., Prakash, R., McAuley, E., . . . Kramer, A. F. (2006). Aerobic exercise training increases brain volume in aging humans. *The Journals of Gerontology Series A: Biological Sciences and Medical Sciences, 61*(11), 1166-1170.

5   Ge, Y., Grossman, R. I., Babb, J. S., Rabin, M. L., Mannon, L. J., & Kolson, D. L. (2002). Age-related total grey matter and white matter changes in normal adult brain. Part 1: Volumetric MR imaging analysis. *American Journal of Neuroradiology, 23*, 1327-1333.

6   Peters, R. (2006). Ageing and the brain. *Postgraduate Medical Journal, 82*(964), 84-88.

7   Zhu, N., Jacobs, D. R., Schreiner, P. J., Launer, L. J., Whitmer, R. A., Sidney, S., . . . Bryan, R. N. (2015). Cardiorespiratory fitness and brain volume and white matter integrity: The CARDIA Study. *Neurology, 84*(23), 2347-2353.

8   Centers for Disease Control and Prevention. (2015, June 04). *How much physical activity do adults need?* Retrieved from http://www.cdc.gov/physicalactivity/basics/adults/

9   Centers for Disease Control and Prevention. (2015, June 04). *How much physical activity do adults need?* Retrieved from http://www.cdc.gov/physicalactivity/basics/adults/

10 World Health Organization. (n.d.). *Physical inactivity: A global public health problem.* Retrieved from http://www.who.int/dietphysicalactivity/factsheet_inactivity/en/

11   Finkelstein, E. A., Ruhm, C. J., & Kosa, K. M. (2005). Economic causes and consequences of obesity. *Annual Review of Public Health, 26*(1), 239-257.

12   Bamman, M. (n.d.) General principles of exercise for health and fitness. Retrieved from http://mbamman.huntingdon.edu/SSPE304/PPTs/ch2.ppt

13   Goldhaber, S. Z., & Morrison, R. B. (2002). Pulmonary embolism and deep vein thrombosis. *Circulation, 106*(12), 1436-1438.

14   Lin, F., Parthasarathy, S., Taylor, S. J., Pucci, D., Hendrix, R. W., & Makhsous, M. (2006). Effect of different sitting postures on lung capacity, expiratory flow, and lumbar lordosis. *Archives of Physical Medicine and Rehabilitation, 87*(4), 504-509.

15   Nair, S., Sagar, M., Sollers, J., Consedine, N., & Broadbent, E. (2015). Do slumped and upright postures affect stress responses? A randomized trial. *Health Psychology, 34*(6), 632-641.

16   American Chiropractic Association. (n.d.). *Tips to maintain good posture.* Retrieved from http://www.acatoday.org/Patients/Health-Wellness-Information/Posture

17   National Institute of Neurological Disorders and Stroke. (2014, July). *Brain basics: Understanding sleep.* Retrieved from http://www.ninds.nih.gov/disorders/brain_basics/understanding_sleep.htm

18   Hogenkamp, P. S., Nilsson, E., Nilsson, V. C., Chapman, C. D., Vogel, H., Lundberg, L. S., Zarei, S., Cedernaes, J., Rangtell, F. H., Broman, J. E., Dickson, S. L., Brunstrom, J. M., Benedict, C., Schioth, H. B. (2013) Acute sleep deprivation increases portion size and affects food choice in young men. *Psychoneuroendocrinology, 38*(9), 1668-1674.

19   Coren, S. (1996). Daylight savings time and traffic accidents. *New England Journal of Medicine, 334*(14), 924-925.

20   Janszky, I., Ahnve, S., Ljung, R., Mukamal, K. J., Gautam, S., Wallentin, L., & Stenestrand, U. (2012). Daylight saving time shifts and incidence of acute myocardial infarction. Swedish Register of Information and Knowledge about Swedish Heart Intensive Care Admissions (RIKS-HIA). *Sleep Medicine, 13*(3), 237-242.

21   Janszky, I., & Ljung, R. (2008). Shifts to and from daylight saving time and incidence of myocardial infarction. *New England Journal of Medicine, 359*(18), 1966-1968.

22   Dawson, D., & Reid, K. (1997). Fatigue, alcohol and performance impairment. *Nature, 388*, 235-237.

23   Banks, S., & Dinges, D. F. (2007). Behavioral and physiological consequences of sleep restriction. *Journal of Clinical Sleep Medicine, 3*(5), 519-528.

24 Gangswisch, J. E., Heymsfield, S. B., Boden-Albala, B., Bujis, R. M., Kreier, F., Pickering, T. G., . . . Malaspina, D. (2007). Sleep duration as a risk factor for diabetes incidence in a large US sample. *Sleep, 30*(12), 1667-1673.

25 Gangswisch, J. E., Malaspina, D., Babiss, L. A., Opler, M. G., Posner, K., Shen, S., . . . Ginsberg, H. N. (2010). Short sleep duration as a risk factor for hypercholesterolemia: Analyses of the national longitudinal study of adolescent health. *Sleep, 33*(7), 956-961.

26 Goel, N., & Dinges, D. F. (2011). Behavioral and genetic markers of sleepiness. *Journal of Clinical Sleep Medicine, S7*(5).

27 National Sleep Foundation. (2015). *National Sleep Foundation recommends new sleep times.* Retrieved from https://sleepfoundation.org/media-center/press-release/national-sleep-foundation-recommends-new-sleep-times

28 Horne, J., Anderson, C., & Platten, C. (2008). Sleep extension versus nap or coffee, within the context of 'sleep debt'. *Journal of Sleep Research, 17*(4), 432-436.

29 Brooks, A., & Lack, L. (2009). A brief afternoon nap following nocturnal sleep restriction: Which nap duration is most recuperative? *Sleep, 29*(6), 831-840.

30 Brooks, A., & Lack, L. (2009). A brief afternoon nap following nocturnal sleep restriction: Which nap duration is most recuperative? *Sleep, 29*(6), 831-840.

31 Walker, M. P., & Stickgold, R. (2004). Sleep-dependent learning and memory consolidation. *Neuron, 44*(1), 121-133.

32 Walker, M. P., & Stickgold, R. (2004). Sleep-dependent learning and memory consolidation. *Neuron, 44*(1), 121-133.

33 Heid, M. (2014, August 27). *What's the ideal bed time?* Retrieved from http://time.com/3183183/you-asked-whats-the-ideal-time-to-go-to-sleep/

34 Sroykham, W., & Wongsawat, Y. (2013). *Effects of LED-backlit computer screen and emotional self-regulation on human melatonin production.* 2013 35th Annual International Conference of the IEEE Engineering in Medicine and Biology Society (EMBC).

35 Yetish, G., Kaplan, H., Gurven, M., Wood, B., Pontzer, H., Manger, P., . . . Siegel, J. (2015). Natural sleep and its seasonal variations in three pre-industrial societies. *Current Biology, 25*(21), 2862-2868.

36 Ekirch, A. R. (2001). Sleep we have lost: Pre-industrial slumber in the British Isles. *The American Historical Review, 106*(2), 343.

37   Wehr, T. A. (1992). In short photoperiods, human sleep is biphasic. *Journal of Sleep Research, 1*(2), 103-107.

PART III

NOURISH

"The food you eat can be either the safest and most powerful form of medicine or the slowest form of poison."
—Ann Wigmore

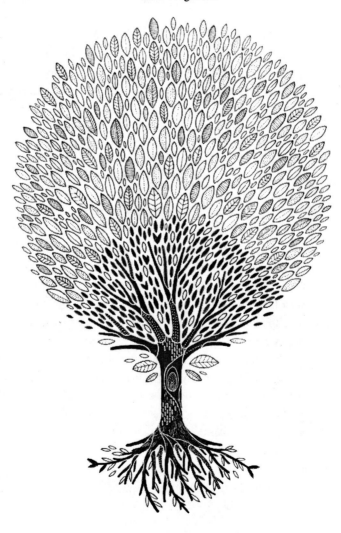

Chapter 9

Sustain Your Body

Our info-saturated world often influences our eating decisions about what, when and how we should eat. Unfortunately, not all advice from the outside world is created equal, and the obsession over finding the perfect diet has caused many of us to lose touch with the valuable information coming directly from our bodies and our natural environments.

Contrary to common practice, eating healthy is not about looking for everything "nonfat," going on extreme diets claimed to "detox" our insides, counting calories, or becoming obsessive over how many grams of fiber or other nutrients we are getting. Rather, it is about reconnecting with our bodies, understanding how our natural environment cycles nutrients to us, and rediscovering the meaningful pleasures of eating well.

Eat Well to Live Well

Physical health depends to a great degree on what you feed your body. And adopting healthy eating habits is not just for middle-aged adults who want to prevent illnesses or delay the aging process. Eating well is for everybody: kids and teenagers who need optimal nutrients for healthy physical and mental development; young adults who need lots of energy to stay productive every day in order to handle our fast-paced modern world; and aging grandparents who want to achieve a healthy longevity so they can keep up with their grandchildren.

We often overlook the fact that many chronic illnesses in middle age are actually the result of long-term exposure to unhealthy lifestyles from one's younger years, including a lack of regular physical activity and diets high in unhealthy fats, sugars, and salt.[1] Because their bodies are able to recover more easily, children and young adults may not immediately feel the direct impact of unhealthy lifestyles. But this does not make their actions—or the subsequent consequences of these actions—harmless.

Eating well, no matter what stage of life you are in, can have amazing short-term and long-term benefits for you. After all, good health is not just the mere absence of disease or infirmity, but "a state of complete physical, mental, and social well-being."[2]

As you begin to adopt a more holistically healthy diet, remember that just like any other lifestyle change, it will be a work in progress. It will take time, but it will be a worthy investment that can help to keep your mind, body, and environment healthy for as long as you live.

The Search for One Ideal Diet Is Over

While dietary guidelines attempt to illustrate the 'perfect diet' for the average person, hardly any individual is an average person. As Denise Minger emphasizes in her info-rich, thought-provoking book, *Death by Food Pyramid*, we all have different genes that result in our bodies reacting differently to what we eat.[3] Some of those differences include: how our saliva contents help us process starch, how we respond to dietary cholesterol and saturated fats, how capable our bodies are of handling vegetarian or vegan diets, etc. You may also have a family history of certain diseases you need to consider when determining what you eat. Because all of our bodies are different, the so-called "perfect diet" for you may not be the one for me, and the perfect "average" diet may not work for either of us.

To complicate matters further, even the most knowledgeable health experts do not fully understand how chemicals within whole foods interact with one another or react with each other inside our bodies. Remember the triangle food pyramid with carbohydrates at the very bottom? Well, not all carbohydrates are created equal. For example, *refined carbohydrates* have been shown to be harmful to health, while carbohydrates from whole grains are deemed to be good for you.[4]

And the fat-free or low-fat diets that are supposed to fight obesity and other diseases? It turns out that the prevalence of obesity has actually increased at the same time dietary fat intake has decreased, suggesting that cutting down on fat alone is not an adequate solution for better health.[5] Plus, not all fats are created equal, either. While trans fats (typically found in processed foods) are detrimental to health, high-quality unsaturated fats from avocados, olive oil, canola oil, nuts, fatty fish, etc., are vital to good health.

Furthermore, numerous studies challenge the notion that the previously demonized saturated fats are harmful to health.[6-9] Have you heard of the *full-fat paradox*? Various studies have shown that full-fat dairy (rich in saturated fats) is actually associated with a *lower* risk of obesity and levels of body fat.[10,11] Although the reason is still unclear, these findings reveal the complex nature of nutrition itself. There is so much we—even our scientific communities—have yet to learn.

So, how can we begin to eat healthier if our understanding of individual nutrients continues to change? Well, since we rarely ever eat any one nutrient alone (i.e., other than when we take synthetic supplements), perhaps we shouldn't obsessively count individual nutrients or calories to match the recommended daily amounts. After all, everyone's lifestyle is different, and everyone's body processes food differently; two bananas grown in different soils can differ in their nutritional contents; not all calories are created equal; and our current knowledge of nutrition is not absolute. Alas, the search for one ideal diet for all is fundamentally flawed. While dietary guidelines are certainly important references, we must also understand what our unique bodies need, where our nutrients come from within our natural environments, and what our surrounding landscapes can provide.

Remember the Purpose of Eating

Recent trends popularize various special diets. Some of these trends are based on religious beliefs; others are followed for health, moral, or ecological reasons. While you absolutely have a right to make your own personal decision regarding your diet, remember that the true purpose of eating, first and foremost, is to nourish your body. That said, there are certainly healthy ways to follow each of these special diets if you know your body well, understand its needs, and are knowledgeable about how to best balance your diet to optimize nutrition.

No matter what your diet looks like, it must provide you with sufficient amounts of your key macronutrients (protein, fats, carbohydrates) and micronutrients (minerals, vitamins, and phytochemicals).[12,13] To accomplish this without needing to isolate and count individual nutrients, ChooseMyPlate.gov from the U.S. Department of Agriculture (USDA) recommends filling your plate with 50% fruits and vegetables, 25% protein-rich foods, and 25% whole grains.[14] However, keep in mind that this is just a rough guideline, and you should adjust these amounts according to your individual lifestyle and preferences, as well as what you feel works best for your body.

Ellen Passov, a Registered Dietitian Nutritionist based in New York, suggests that healthy people should include all food groups in their diets unless there is a particular reason why they are unable to. These food groups typically comprise fruits, vegetables, grains, protein-rich foods, and dairy (which includes calcium-fortified alternative milks).[15] Since certain nutrients are particular to each food group, the more restrictive your diet, the more personal homework you will need to do about how to include the nutrients you might be missing.

While taking daily multivitamin supplements may sound like the way to make up for potentially missed nutrients, research has actually shown that *untargeted* vitamin supplements offer little or nothing in terms of health benefits for well-nourished adults, and that high doses of certain vitamins can even cause harm.[16] Therefore, if you have special dietary restrictions, speak with your dietician to see how you can best supplement your specific diet.

In general, however, aim to get most of your nutrients from whole foods and to get your foods from a variety of sources. After all, the more variety your diet has, the more balanced your nutritional profile will be, and the less you will have to worry about nutrient deficiencies!

Question Food Labels

"Detoxing" is all the hype these days—juicing, water-fasting, you name it. Our food industry has been filled with (expensive) products claiming to "cleanse" our bodies. Unfortunately, there is no such thing as a "cleansing" or "detoxing" food product. Sense About Science, a British nonprofit organization with a database of more than 6,000 scientists aiming to promote public understanding of science, noted: "The multimillion [dollar] detox industry sells products with little evidence to support their use. These products trade on claims about the body which are often wrong and can be dangerous." [17] Unfortunately, the idea that a special meal or beverage can flush out toxins from our bodies is just a pure marketing ploy and completely underestimates the amazing functions our bodies are capable of.

Meet your liver, kidneys, lungs, gastrointestinal tract, and skin—vital organs that have been detoxifying your body since day one. It is their job to keep the good stuff in and flush the bad stuff out. Therefore, in essence, the "detox" labels on our food products carry no meaningful value on their own. Your best way to detox is simply to keep your entire body healthy so your organs can function properly.

That said, consuming "detox" products that are indeed rich in nutrients poses no threat (and can even be beneficial) to your health. However, instead of being lured by any *unregulated* food labels that don't really mean anything scientifically ("natural," "detox," "premium," "superfood," etc.), always check the list of ingredients as your most factual way to determine whether or not something truly contains nutritious, wholesome ingredients.

If you ever decide to test out any "cleansing" products or diets to reset your palate or begin a clean slate for healthy eating habits, just do so in moderation. And keep in mind that you can get the benefits out of "cleanses" without the potential harms simply by drinking more water, cutting out junk food, and incorporating more whole fruits and vegetables into your diet. After all, your best way to efficiently absorb nutrients and expel toxins is to keep your body holistically healthy so your organs can function properly; that is, by taking care of your inner well-being, getting regular physical activity, obtaining sufficient quality sleep, *regularly* eating a balanced diet dominated by whole foods, staying hydrated, and minimizing your intake of unhealthy substances (alcohol, drugs, junk food, etc.).

Master Your Body's Language

There is contradictory advice on how many meals a day is best—three, five, or even ten? How many calories should a meal contain—300, 500, or more? The truth is, there is no one magic number for everyone, because everyone's body is different. Instead of relying solely on external portion guidelines, try to get back in tune with the important cues coming directly from your own body.

Unfortunately, all of the junk food out there, the oversized portions served at restaurants, and even the guidelines for the "average person" have caused many of us to lose touch with our bodily signals. However, we all are born with the innate ability to detect hunger, thirst, and fullness. Thus, if we practice mindful eating, we will better understand how much our bodies truly need for any one particular sitting. If you feel completely out of touch with your sense of hunger or fullness, however, seek guidance from a health professional.

Since it takes 15-20 minutes for your brain to recognize that you are full, you will often reach satiety before you actually feel it.[18] Therefore, if you eat until you *feel* full, you may already be eating too much for that one sitting. Overeating not only contributes to weight gain but also feels uncomfortable, exerts stress on your body, and hinders healthy digestion. Instead of gobbling everything down and eating until you hit a "food coma," eat slowly, chew your food well, drink water with your meals, check in with your body every so often to see how full you are, and stop once you feel a little pressure in your stomach. It may take some time to turn this into a natural habit, but it will become second nature over time.

The Okinawan people of Japan have a life expectancy among the highest in the world, and they also have significantly lower death rates from cerebral vascular disease, malignancy, and heart disease compared to the rest of Japan.[19] One isolated difference in their lifestyle from the rest of the country is their rule of healthy eating called *hara hachi bu,* which translates to "eat until you are 80% full." For example, calorie intake by their schoolchildren was just 62% of the "recommended" intake for Japan, while calorie intake for their adults was 20% less than the Japanese national average.[20] Although genetics and other lifestyle factors may be at play, even Okinawans who moved to other islands had higher mortality rates than those who remained! This suggests that their lower risks for illnesses may be attributed to their culture and habit of eating moderately.

Research studies have also found that dietary calorie restriction decreased mortality rates in various tested animals, suggesting that the same effect may apply to humans.[21,22] This does not imply that we should starve ourselves, but that eating until we are *moderately* satisfied, rather than too full, can be beneficial to our health over time.

If you sometimes accidentally overeat, there is no need to feel guilty about it; few are capable of perfect eating habits. Instead, just focus on going back to being in tune with your bodily signals again as soon as possible—preferably by the time the next meal rolls around.

Because caloric guidelines are simply averages, and not all calories are processed in the same way by our bodies, *mindful eating* is a healthier, more accurate, and more natural alternative to counting calories. As long as you sleep well and minimize empty calories, junk food and sugary drinks, your body will know better than anyone when it is satisfied or needs more.

A Recharged Morning and a Restful Night

It goes without saying that we need to eat in order to fuel our bodies. However, it turns out that the timing of our meals, particularly our breakfasts and dinners, can also have important health implications for us.

Researcher Leah Cahill concluded from her study in 2013 that skipping breakfast or eating late at night may lead to obesity, high blood pressure, high cholesterol, and diabetes, thus increasing one's risk for coronary heart disease.[23] This makes sense; your body must be renourished with the proper nutrition it needs for a healthy start in the morning.

In fact, eating breakfast can improve short-term memory and attention; in a research study, students who ate breakfast tended to perform better in school than those who did not.[24] Since you are literally putting your body on an overnight fast when you sleep, you do not want to leave your body in prolonged starvation mode by missing breakfast. The resulting stress will likely make you crave unhealthy snacks later in the day.

While you should certainly not be grumbling with hunger at night, you should also not feel burdened by a big meal when you are about to sleep. Because your body needs time to digest your food, eating huge meals right before sleeping can keep your stomach from getting the proper rest it needs overnight. Moreover, lying down on a full stomach can also cause acid reflux, which can damage your esophagus. If you are kept awake from hunger, just eat something light. However, if you are uncomfortably full at bedtime, make sure you walk around a little before lying down.

If properly scheduling your morning and evening meals can contribute to your long-term health, maybe it will be worth planning ahead to ensure you have enough time to have a healthy breakfast in the morning and avoid heavy late-night meals right before going to bed!

Chapter Summary

Eat Well to Live Well

Because many chronic illnesses develop over years or even decades, the importance of a healthy diet is often overlooked. No matter your age or health status, eating well will provide you with both immediate and long-term benefits.

The Search for One Ideal Diet Is Over

Because of the differences among our bodies and the infinite ways in which chemicals in our foods can interact with one another and within our bodies, there is no such thing as one ideal diet. Instead, to find **your** unique and ideal diet, you will have to consider not only dietary guideline recommendations and your personal beliefs but also your own body's condition and what your natural environment can sustainably provide you.

Remember the Purpose of Eating

No matter what special diet you might have, remember that the primary purpose of eating is to nourish your body so that you can function at your maximum potential. Because there are nutrients particular to each food group, the more restrictive your diet, the more personal homework you will need to do on how to best supplement your diet to prevent nutritional deficiencies.

Question Food Labels

The best way for you to help your body detox is to live a holistically healthy lifestyle so that your organs can function properly. Question any unregulated food labels ("detox," "superfood," "all natural," etc.) when you shop, and always check a product's list of ingredients to determine whether or not it truly contains nutritious, wholesome ingredients.

Master Your Body's Language

To best understand how much to eat per meal, get back in touch with your body's own hunger and fullness signals. So long as you sleep well and minimize junk food, sugary drinks, and processed foods that may throw off your hunger cues, your body will know better than anyone when it needs more or when it is satisfied. To prevent overeating, chew your food well and slowly, drink water with your meals, check in frequently to see how full you are, and stop once you feel some pressure exerted in your stomach.

Chapter Summary (Cont'd)

A Recharged Morning and a Restful Night

To get a healthy start to your day, do not forget to break your overnight fast in the morning! And, to ensure a restful sleep at night, avoid big meals right before going to sleep. Have something light if you are being kept awake by hunger, or walk around a little before lying down if you feel too full.

Chapter 10

Nourish Your Body

By definition, *food* is any *nutritious substance* people or animals eat or drink to *maintain life* and *growth*. However, many things we eat today not only lack nutrition, but also may harm our health! Start questioning whether what you are eating is even considered "food," and definitely try to keep anything that is not to a minimum in your diet.

Dump the Junk!

From white rice to white bread, candies, cookies, and cakes, the modern diet is rather heavy in processed foods. While most processed foods do come from natural whole foods, many of their original nutrients are lost during the production process. For example, the bran and germ of a whole grain are extracted when producing refined carbohydrates. This process removes not only the fiber but also much of the grain's nutritional value, including B-complex vitamins, healthy oils, phytonutrients, and fat-soluble vitamins.

To make matters worse, the more processed a food is, the more added sugars, salt, and unhealthy fats there probably are. While we are hardwired through evolution to crave fatty and sweet foods for high energy and efficiency, studies have already linked diets high in added sugar, salt, trans fats, and refined carbohydrates to obesity, tooth decay, and possibly diabetes, high blood pressure, heart disease, anemia, skin problems, kidney disease, and cancer.[25-29] It's not that our evolutionary instincts are wrong, only that junk foods—rich in unhealthy fats and added sugars—have become too readily available to us. Plus, processed and refined foods also have high *glycemic index values*; that is, the carbohydrates in these foods get absorbed quickly into our bodies and spike up our blood sugar more rapidly. Regular consumption of these foods, then, would pose a big concern for diabetics and for anyone's general, long-term health.

Another type of harmful substance known as Advanced Glycation End-products (AGEs) proliferates especially when foods are processed, fried, or dry-cooked at high temperatures. Unfortunately, long-term exposure to these substances may increase the risk of diabetes, heart disease, kidney disease, and other chronic illnesses.[30]

As you can see, the more processed a food is, the more original good stuff it loses and the more undesirable substances it gains. Therefore, not only are most junk foods lacking in nutrients, but they are actually *harmful* to your body! This doesn't quite sound like what food is supposed to do for us.

Thankfully, it does not require much extra time and effort to substitute processed foods with healthier alternatives. For example, substituting whole fruits for snack bars or cookies rich in added sugars and trans fats takes no effort at all. To save time making fresh home-cooked meals, you can also use precut frozen vegetables, which have similar or sometimes even more nutrients than fresh produce because they are "flash-frozen" right after being harvested at their peak ripeness.[31,32]

When you begin to cut out processed foods, you might still have sudden cravings for junk food. This is because junk food is like a drug for your brain—it's specially formulated to be addictive! Therefore, your first few weeks of cutting down on processed foods may require more conscious effort. After a while, however, so long as your diet is dominated by a variety of whole foods, don't be too hard on yourself and give yourself the freedom to eat whatever you like, sometimes—in moderation.

Eat Whole to Be Whole

The complexity of nutrition and the human body goes beyond our current knowledge. And there is much more to nutrition than just the proteins, fats, carbs, vitamins, minerals, and fiber contents we tend to focus on. This is because *whole foods*—ones that are processed minimally (see Table 10-1)—contain many health-boosting chemicals within them that we do not yet fully understand. For example, vegetables and fruits contain numerous types of *phytochemicals*—nonessential nutrients present in whole plant foods—within them. There are tens of thousands of them that we already know exist, but there are even more we have yet to discover. Although we still need to learn about the biological effects of all the phytochemicals out there, we do know that they have amazing health-boosting properties that can help protect us against diseases.

While we typically examine the effects of only independent nutrients, the chemicals within whole foods can interact with one another to produce biological consequences different from those produced in singular nutrients—a concept called "food synergy." The same can happen for paired-together nutrients found in different whole foods as well. As Laura Rosenberg, a Registered Dietitian, chef and culinary educator at the Natural Gourmet Institute, noted, "Whole foods are *more* than the sum of their parts."[33] So, counting milligrams of nutrients, fiber and calories independently does not end up telling the whole story!

Table 10-1. Some Whole Foods and Their Processed Counterparts

Whole Foods	Their Processed Counterparts
Fresh fruits, frozen fruits	Fruit juices, fruit snacks, fruit pies
Fresh vegetables, frozen vegetables	Vegetable juice, vegetable chips, fries
Fresh, lean meats and fish, eggs	Hot dogs, chicken nuggets, deli meats
Plain yogurt, fresh milk	Sweetened yogurt, flavored milk, cheesecake, desserts
Whole grains such as brown rice, wild rice, whole oats, quinoa, couscous, etc.	White rice, white bread, pie crust, frozen meals, baked goods

One example of food synergy is how vitamin C helps your body to better absorb nonheme iron.[34,35] While our bodies are generally capable of efficiently absorbing iron from meats (which contain both heme iron and nonheme iron), they are less capable of absorbing iron from plants and other iron-fortified foods (which contain only nonheme iron). Therefore, eating dark leafy greens (rich in nonheme iron) simultaneously with tomatoes (rich in vitamin C) can help you to better absorb the iron than if you were to just eat the greens by themselves. Similarly, adding black pepper to your meals can help to improve your body's absorption of various types of nutrients from your food.[36-38]

Think about how many endless possibilities there are for potential health-boosting chemical interactions between all of the nutrients out there—chemicals within whole foods and chemicals within different foods when paired together. It is truly mind-blowing. The bottom line is, our bodies thrive on a diversity of (whole) food sources, just as our planet thrives with biodiversity.

What does this mean when it comes to selecting your meals? If you have a choice between a colorful, mixed salad versus a bowl of kale, the first option is likely your more nutritionally balanced choice. Similarly, choosing to get your protein from a wide variety of sources—switching up between grass-fed meat, pastured dairy, seafood, poultry, nuts, seeds, and legumes—is better than just getting your protein from only steak or only tofu. This does not mean that you need to eat 10 types of vegetables and get your protein from 10 different sources within every single meal, but you should seek variety within individual meals or at least over the course of several meals.

Water, Water Everywhere, but Don't Forget to Drink

What is water? It is the most abundant liquid on earth. In solid form (ice) and liquid form, it covers about 70% of the earth's surface. Chemically, water is a compound of hydrogen and oxygen whose formula is H_2O. Water serves both as a heat-transfer medium (e.g., ice for cooling and steam for heating) and as a temperature regulator (the water in lakes and oceans helps regulate the climate). Finally, and most important, other than air, food, and sunlight, water is the most essential element of life. Humans need it to survive.

Despite the endless beverage options in supermarkets and convenient stores, the most natural and healthiest way to hydrate is still with water (plain water, infused water, or herbal teas). This is because many artificial drinks and sodas contain excessive amounts of sugars and sodium. And while fruit juices may be healthier alternatives to artificial drinks, research suggests that it is more nutritious to eat your fruits and vegetables whole rather than drinking their juice.[39] In fact, eating more whole fruits was significantly associated with a lower risk of type 2 diabetes, while greater consumption of fruit juices was associated with a *higher* risk of type 2 diabetes.[40,41] Since juicing a fruit or vegetable removes some or all of its fiber, drinking juice elevates blood sugar much more rapidly than eating whole fruits and vegetables.

Also, juices can be high in calories but not very filling. For example, one cup of chopped apples is around 60 calories, while one cup of fresh apple juice is around 110. While it may take you a couple of minutes to chomp down that cup of refreshing apple slices, it could take you less than 10 seconds to gulp down that cup of juice without even feeling satisfied. This is not to say that you should stop drinking juice completely, because drinking juice can be a quick way to boost energy and increase your intake of fruits and vegetables. However, if you have the time and option, choose to consume the majority of your fruits and vegetables whole. Their high-fiber contents can help to improve digestion and make you feel fuller longer, thus preventing you from overeating! As a bonus, you will also generate less plastic juice container waste.

Cheers to Good Health

Many of us (over the legal drinking age) enjoy having alcoholic beverages here and there, whether during social events, alongside meals, or just in the comforts of our homes. However, there are certain things to keep in mind when we choose to get loose with some booze. Yes, we all want to have fun, and the buzz we get from alcohol can spice up our lives. But with more informed decisions, we will stay healthy longer and then have more time to have more fun! For starters, check the following table to see what level of drinker you are (see Table 10-2).

Table 10-2. Levels of Alcohol Drinkers[42]

Level	For Women	For Men
Moderate drinker	1 drink per day	2 drinks per day
Drinker at risk for alcohol use disorder	More than 3 drinks a day or 7 per week	More than 4 drinks a day or 14 per week
Binge drinker	4+ drinks in 2 hours	5+ drinks in 2 hours
Heavy drinker	5+ drinks on each occasion for each of 5+ days in the last month	

There is no use denying that alcohol is poison to our bodies. If you do not drink at all or are a moderate drinker, your risk of damaging your body with alcohol consumption is pretty low. However, for those who drink more than moderately, remember that the negative health effects of alcohol consumption may not necessarily occur overnight but rather through long-term and consistent abuse. While what is considered "moderate" may differ for every individual, the more often you drink past your body's signals for you to stop (headaches, dizziness, impaired judgments, losing control over your body, nausea, etc.), the higher your risk for developing chronic diseases. These potential illnesses include various types of cancers, cirrhosis of the liver, anemia, cardiovascular diseases, dementia, seizures, high blood pressure, infectious diseases, and nerve damage, among many others. Moreover, some alcoholic beverages may also be contaminated with heavy metals; a study found relatively high levels of potentially hazardous heavy metal ions in red and white wines from various countries, which may contribute to chronic inflammatory diseases, premature aging, and disruption of normal cell and tissue function.[43]

Even if you do not drink regularly, overdrinking during any one episode can increase your risks for impaired cognitive functions, disrupted sleep cycles, hangovers, brain damage, and alcohol poisoning. And although alcohol in moderation, like a glass of red wine every day, may be good for cardiovascular health, keep in mind that even moderate alcohol intake is associated with increased risks for illnesses, violence, drowning, injuries, and car accidents.[44]

As you can see, alcohol consumption is associated with numerous health risks. However, as long as you have the proper knowledge on how to drink safely and responsibly, you do not have to be too restrictive. To prevent chronic illnesses and short-term damages without completely cutting out alcohol, celebrate occasionally, but in moderation, and stop drinking when your body signals you to (when you get headaches, feel nauseous, etc.)!

Chapter Summary

Dump the Junk!

Not only are most processed or junk foods lacking in nutrients, but they even contain substances harmful to health. Moreover, because they are like drugs to our brain, it is easy to become addicted to them. So, try to slowly cut down on the amount of processed foods in your diet, and know that it will take a few weeks of conscious effort to do so. After your diet becomes dominated by whole foods, however, don't be too hard on yourself and give yourself the freedom to indulge (moderately) in whatever you like once in a while.

Eat Whole to Be Whole

Nutrition is extremely complex, because chemicals within whole foods can interact to have biological consequences not yet fully understood by us. What we do know, however, is that these chemical interactions are beneficial to our health and that whole foods end up being more than the sum of their parts. To optimize nutrition, eat a variety of whole foods.

Water, Water Everywhere, but Don't Forget to Drink

Staying hydrated is vital for the healthy functioning of every organ within your body. Although fruit and vegetable juices are healthier alternatives to artificial drinks, much of the important fiber contents, which help slow down your body's absorption of their sugars, are lost. While they may be great for quick boosts of energy and a way to increase your intake of fruits and vegetables, try to eat the majority of your fruits and veggies whole and hydrate mostly with plain water, infused water, or herbal teas!

Cheers to Good Health

We all like to have fun and have a drink once in a while. However, keep in mind that the effects of risky alcohol use may not surface overnight but through long-term, chronic abuse. Therefore, drinking responsibly now can help you to decrease your risks of short-term damage and long-term chronic illness.

Chapter 11

Nourish Your Food

You might be saying right about now, "I get the point: Just eat more whole foods because they are more nutritious." But bear with me, because the story goes on, and there is more to healthy eating than just choosing to eat your foods whole. To complicate matters a little, I must tell you that not all whole foods are created equal.

We get our nutrients from our food, but where do they get *theirs* from? Like us, our foods absorb nutrients from what they eat or what environments they are raised in. If a cow grows up eating nutritious grasses (as opposed to corn or grain, which is unnatural to its digestive system), it will be healthier, and its meat will be more nutritious, too. If an apple grows up in healthy soil (as opposed to a nutrient-depleted one), it will have absorbed more nutrients and be more nutritious as well.

When we examine where our nutrients come from, it becomes clear that if we want to be healthy, we *need* our food to be healthy first. Therefore, we must support agricultural systems that not only produce food but also aim to produce food in healthful ways.

Beauty from Within

On a Monday evening many years ago, I sat down next to my grandfather, who was reminiscing about his childhood growing up on a farm in Taiwan. All of their farming was done by hand with no additional chemicals.

"What about the pests?" I asked.

"They were there," he said calmly, as if it were not a big deal. "Sometimes we picked them by hand, sometimes their natural predators preyed on them, and sometimes they were still there. It was normal to have a few holes or bruises on our harvested vegetables, but it was fine. They were perfectly edible. What mattered most was just that our lands were healthy and productive, which would better ensure food security for us for many years to come."

And then my grandfather's words struck me. Have we been too shallow by valuing the *looks* of our produce more than the way it was raised? Instead of judging our food purely based on its physical properties (looks, texture, smell, etc.), we need to begin seeking beauty on a deeper level. Instead of focusing only on the outcomes, we will need to shed light on the *processes* of our food production.

Although chemical-intensive farming dominates many agricultural systems in the world today, sustainable farming practices combining ancient knowledge, traditional farming techniques and new technology are on the rise. These sustainable practices include (but are not limited to) intercropping, increasing crop diversity, and using cover crops, crop rotation, or mechanical, manual, and biological pest control methods. Meanwhile, conventional farming continues to rely on cheap chemicals to maximize current yields. Is it too strong a statement to say that conventional farming is like a drug-addicted form of farming?

For the sake of our own health and food security, we need to support small-scale, sustainable farms that use deep understandings of the environment, together with the knowledge of farming practices that work *in harmony* with the rhythms of nature rather than against them. One way to find these farms is to ask around at your local farmers' markets. Talk to your farmers and get to know how they grow and produce the foods that they sell. When this is not possible, however, looking for the organic label may be your next best choice. Although organic certifications are not perfect and may vary in their standards, their aim to encourage the protection of human and environmental health is still crucial for long-term sustainability.

Revive Our Silent Springs

When we shop for our groceries, it is natural to ponder whether paying a few cents or dollars extra for higher-quality produce is worth the money. But when we come to see that these decisions can and will directly affect us, our farmers, our drinking water, our clean air, and our entire ecosystem, the answer becomes quite clear: Choosing food produced responsibly is a survival *need*. Although we may not always have the access or budget, every time we pick sustainably grown food over its conventional counterparts counts. There is no need to brood over the times when you have no choice, but it is important to realize that when you do, you can make a meaningful difference.

Lack of access to clean water is an increasingly prominent problem today, and we ourselves are the culprits. When we support farms that use and release toxic chemicals into our environment, we are just increasing our own health risks. While our current water purification systems are by and large successful at filtering out targeted contaminants, unspecified toxic chemicals from fertilizers, insecticides, industry wastes, or even petroleum leaks may pass through, making our "purified" water not as pure as we had imagined. Unfortunately, in the United States, there have already been numerous cases of unsafe levels of toxins found in tap water deemed "safe to drink" (see Chapter 15). If we want to minimize the amount of toxins lurking in our drinking water, we can help to target the problem at its roots by supporting agricultural practices that make it their mission to cut down on pollution and the use of toxic chemicals.

An immediate and evident benefit from eating organic foods is that it can dramatically decrease our exposures to organosphosphate pesticides—a type of synthetic pesticide that is highly toxic to wildlife and humans—often used in conventional farming.[45,46] However, eating organic foods actually does not eliminate our exposures to all types of pesticides. This is because organic farming still permits the use of *natural* pesticides when other pest control methods (i.e., mechanical or biological pest control) are ineffective. Unfortunately, natural pesticides can be toxic as well.

Pesticides, whether natural or synthetic, are made to harm insects, birds, and sometimes even mammals—we are mammals, too! Exposures to pesticides have been linked to various acute and chronic health problems for humans, especially for children; this suggests that we should keep pesticide use to a bare minimum.[47-51]

At the moment, there is little to no official way to know whether or not pesticides were used in growing your food (unless you personally know your farmer). However, I encourage you to still ask your farmers or grocers about the use of pesticides in the food they sell. Although they are not obligated to tell you the truth—and your grocers might not know—at least you will initiate an important dialogue and encourage the production of more pesticide-free (or "nonsprayed") produce in the future!

Even with the problems pertaining to agrochemicals aside, supporting responsible agricultural practices is not merely about decreasing our health risks but also about improving our nutrition and well-being. According to *Food is Medicine,* an info-rich book that draws upon hundreds, if not thousands, of research studies on food and nutrition, "There is accumulating scientific data portraying nonsprayed organic fruits and vegetables, generally grown in nutrient-replenished soil, to be *far superior nutrient sources* than chemically saturated, commercially grown varieties harvested from virtual wastelands."[52]

Although certain short-term studies argue against this statement, whether or not all organic produce necessarily is more nutritious than all conventional produce does not change the way our natural world functions: *Healthier ecosys-*

tems will still be able to sustain healthier living species. Therefore, instead of focusing on any particular study, we should be looking at the bigger and broader question here: What is healthier and more sustainable for our planet—and, consequently, for ourselves?

Lower Yield; Not a Big Deal

One common argument against organic farming is that it generally produces fewer yields than conventional farming. However, organic farming technology is constantly improving, and the yields for certain crops have already caught up to those of conventional agriculture. But is yield even the most important factor to consider? Many say that we cannot afford to have lower yields because of world hunger problems. But allow me to enlighten you with the following facts about hunger and food waste:

- Nearly one-third of food produced in the world is wasted every year.[53]

- When food rots in landfills, it becomes a significant source of methane—a potent greenhouse gas with 21 times the global warming potential of carbon dioxide.[54]

- Every single hungry individual in the world (about one billion people) could be lifted out of malnutrition on less than a quarter of the food wasted in the United States, United Kingdom, and Europe. [55]

Evidently, our current global food supply is already more than enough to feed the entire world. This shows that today's world hunger problem stems *not* from a lack of food production; instead, it is a systemic issue resulting from skewed distribution, unsound politics, and wasteful choices. Improving yield certainly can be beneficial, since it would lead to less overall land usage dedicated to food production. However, doing so at the cost of damaging our ecosystem, a common result of conventional farming, is not nearly as desirable as improving yield through better soil and water management practices, the aims of organic farming. Therefore, quantity is not nearly as important as the quality of food production, and it should not be a primary concern that organic farming sometimes produces fewer yields for certain crops.

To help address food waste and world hunger, we must push for supporting legislations that improve distribution and rechannel wasted yet still edible food. For us as individuals, we can also help by reducing the amount of food waste we each generate if we:

- Order only as much as we can eat at restaurants;

- Take leftover food at restaurants "to go";

- At home, prioritize consuming those foods with quickly approaching expiration dates;

- Use the "root-to-stalk," "nose-to-tail" methods when cooking (see Chapter 13); and

- Look past the bruises and bumps on fruits and vegetables when we shop for ourselves.

The GMO Nondebate

The concept of selectively breeding animals or crops to pass on desirable genes is not new to science. However, the use of biotechnology to artificially manipulate an organism's genetic makeup (i.e., which is already done to most of our soy and corn today) only became more prominent toward the end of the 20th century. Recently, the U.S. Food and Drug Administration also approved of AquAdvantage Salmon, the first genetically modified food animal.

Genetically modified organisms (GMOs) are generally defined as organisms in which the original genetic material has been altered using engineering techniques to create crops or animals with more desirable traits. Some crops are engineered to produce their own internal pesticides to deter pests. Other crops and animals (such as AquAdvantage Salmon) are made to grow bigger and faster. No matter what their purposes are, however, there remains a great deal of controversy over whether or not to support GMO technology or require mandatory labeling of GMO products.

As consumers, we want to support business practices that improve our health (and the health of our planet) and help us work toward sustainability. So, should we be pro- or anti-GMOs? The answer is neither—for now, anyway.

Although GMOs are often demonized, there is actually little to no scientific evidence suggesting that their consumption directly causes harm to human health. Moreover, since different biotechnology companies engineer their products differently and for varying purposes, the Institute of Medicine and the National Research Council recommended that the safety of modified foods be tested on a case-by-case basis.[56] Therefore, it is unsound logic and science to consider *all* GMOs to be safe or harmful for the short term.

How about for the long term? Unfortunately, this is a tricky question to answer, as we are still in the process of finding out whether or not the widespread, long-term use of GMOs will have undesirable consequences on our entire ecosystem's functioning over time. Thus, we do need to question whether GMOs are necessary or dependable solutions for sustainable food production.

GMO crops are often engineered to naturally deter pests with their built-in pesticides so farmers will not need to use as much toxic agrochemicals. However, because of the ability of living species to adapt to new environments, the pests can develop characteristics that make them immune to these genetically engineered pest deterrents over time. Therefore, these GMOs would become an ineffective, long-term solution for pest control.

Additionally, crops are often engineered to tolerate herbicides so that when farmers spray herbicides to kill off unwanted weeds, the crops will not be harmed during the process. However, some weeds (known as "superweeds") have already developed herbicide-resistant traits, thus leading farmers to use even more toxic chemicals than they did before. Finally, the constant need for farmers to purchase newly patented GMO seeds prevents the farmers from becoming self-reliant.

As you can see, while GMOs may offer appealing temporary solutions to some of the most common challenges food producers regularly face, they have not yet proven to be viable long-term solutions for sustainable food production.

Even though we have already discovered so much about our world through research in the past few decades, we must acknowledge that we are still nowhere close to fully understanding every chemical interaction and every biological process. Unfortunately, our propensity to mass-produce and use products without completely understanding their consequences (continuing toxic chemical pollution from persistent use of DDT pesticides, widespread dioxins pollution from the manufacturing of many consumer products, etc.) has already led us to create deleterious environments for ourselves. Therefore, instead of messing with the incredible ways our planet's ecosystems and living species have been evolving for billions of years, maybe we should first prioritize sustainable food production methods that we already know work *with* the natural ways our ecosystems function.

Science is advancing rapidly, and there is potential for genetic engineering technology to benefit us in some way down the road—if the long-term human and environmental health risks are comprehensively assessed within controlled laboratory settings first. However, because GMO organisms might pass on their modified genes to nearby non-GMO organisms, which then might spread by themselves, we must beware of any unanticipated consequences and irreversible change to the surrounding environment.

So where does this leave us when it comes to making decisions about GMO foods? As a start, we can push for mandatory labeling of GMO products so that we can at least make informed shopping decisions. At the same time, perhaps we should refrain from being strictly pro- or anti-GMOs. Instead, we should focus first on supporting food production methods that work in harmony with nature, such as small-scale organic farming that encourages crop diversity while minimizing the use of toxic chemicals.

Honor Our Farmers

When you eat, do you ever think of your farmer and your food's story—e.g., the journey that apple in your hand undertook from seedling to tree and from tree to fruit, the way it interacted with the land, drinking water from rain, taking in natural sunlight, and standing tall and strong in the face of harsh weather? Do you think of the way your farmer beamed when the season's fruit first appeared, manually irrigated the tree in times of drought, nourished its soil to keep it healthy, protected it from potential pests, and smiled despite hours of sweat and hard work during harvesting?

Regrettably, the thought of our farmers being at the very forefront producing food vital to our survival and taking care of land vital to our planet's health does not even cross the minds of many consumers. Perhaps it is time to honor our farmers. In a world where many people are disconnected from the sources of their food and unaware of how produce is grown, it is clear that we *need* our farmers. And not only that, but we need happy and healthy farmers who are passionate about our land and knowledgeable about how natural ecosystems function. After all, we are entrusting part of our survival and well-being to these humble and diligent workers as they spend their entire lives helping to keep us and our earth home healthy.

A study examining pesticide toxicity among Indonesian farmers concluded: "For farmers in the tropics, fully protective garb is too hot and too costly to maintain; *farmers thus accept illness as a necessity.*"[57] Especially when healthier methods of agriculture already exist, this last statement is really troubling. Even in the United States, farmers and pesticide applicators were found to be at greater risk of accidental mortality as well as hematopoietic and nervous system cancers, compared to other workers.[58]

What's even more disheartening is that rates of mortality and suicide for farmers are among the highest of all occupations.[59-61] Many farmers are in constant debt due to their heavy reliance on new technology and chemicals. In fact, suicide rates among farmers have been correlated with high levels of insecurity and inability to pay off debts from the high costs of seeds, fertilizers, and pesticides, coupled with high interest rates, international competition, and droughts.[62,63] Sadly, in the name of maintaining their livelihoods, many farmers—often with no other choice—work with methods toxic to their mental and physical health, our planet's health, and our health as consumers.

So what can we do to help protect our farmers, our earth home, and ourselves? Going forward, we need to consciously support higher-quality food production that better uses our farmers' knowledge and skills. We can do this by shopping for organic, nonsprayed produce, pastured, high-quality animal products, and food products from *biodynamic farming*—a form of alternative agriculture that treats the farm and its animals, crops, and soil as an ecosystem, excluding the use of artificial agrochemicals. This will not only help keep everyone healthier, it can also make our farmers feel more satisfied with their lives.[64] Because organic and biodynamic farming require less monetary investment, they will make farmers more self-reliant and financially secure. Since we individually no longer grow our own food or take care of the lands that produce our food, we must honor and respect our farmers, and we must especially support the ones who are passionate about protecting our shared environment.

The next time you go grocery shopping, remember the land and the farmers who produced your food. Look past the aromas, textures, and colors of the produce you pick up for a second and think of its entire journey prior to its resting place in your hand. Does it have an inspirational story rooted in the deep knowledge of the farmers who produced it? Or does it more likely have a story involving toxic environments, chemical poisoning, and damaged ecosystems? *This* is what you are paying for and what your money supports.

Old MacDonald, Where's Your Farm?

Back in the day, well before the mass-production of meat, almost all farms resembled something like the well-known Old MacDonald's farm—simple and small-scaled, where animals happily mooed and quacked in open spaces. No injected hormones or antibiotics, no over-populated cages, and no mass-produced, unnatural feed. Since most animal products today are not the same as the *real* ones from healthy animals we used to eat, we must *consciously* seek for quality over quantity in the animal products we consume.

Unfortunately, most meats sold today are either processed or come from mass-produced, factory-farmed livestock. "So what?" you might ask. First, processed meat (deli meat, ham, sausages, etc.), like any other processed food, loses much of its nutritional value, may form harmful substances during its production, and may contain harmful substances added during its processing.

Second, the environmental impact of factory farming is extremely alarming. The livestock sector as a whole produces a shocking 18% of our greenhouse gases, *more* than the amount produced by transportation![65] Many scientists and environmentalists also agree that livestock farming is one of the leading causes of species extinction, ocean dead zones, water pollution, and habitat destruction.[66] Also, the cheaper prices of factory-farmed animal products are simply the results of the higher efficiency that comes with mass production. Disturbingly, that efficiency is managed by cramming large populations of animals in small, crowded spaces; giving them cheap and unnatural food; injecting them with antibiotics to prevent diseases they are more prone to than animals raised naturally; and injecting them with hormones to get more meat out of each animal.

Although red meats of all qualities are often lumped into the same category and perceived to be unhealthy altogether, the distinction between cheap, factory-farmed meats and high-quality, pasture-raised meats is significant. After all, if an animal isn't healthy, how can its meat be healthy? Indeed, various studies have found that meats from grass-fed cows and lambs are leaner and have healthier nutritional profiles than conventional meat; the same applies to dairy products.[67-69] Grass-fed beef also contains more precursors for vitamins A and E, and even several cancer-fighting antioxidants, compared to grain-fed beef.[70]

What this means is that high-quality, grass-fed meat and dairy, though a little pricier, are proven to be healthier than factory-farmed meat and dairy. This should not come as a surprise to anyone, as the same law of nature that makes us healthier by eating more nutritious foods, being more active, and having less stress applies to animals as well. I doubt that you would find eating greasy meat from sickly or antibiotic- and hormone-injected animals very appetizing.

To find higher-quality meat and dairy products, look out for certifications that disclose whether they are grass-fed or organic. While "grass-fed" refers to animals raised grazing outdoors for food (i.e., eating what they are supposed to eat), the USDA organic label for meat and dairy signifies that:

• Livestock must be raised organically on certified organic land.

• Livestock must be 100% fed with certified organic feed.

- No antibiotics were used.

- No growth hormones were used.

- Livestock must have outdoor access to pastures.

Since the certification process can be costly, however, some farms, even if they meet the same high standards, may choose not to obtain any certifications to keep their costs down. To find these farms, ask around at your local farmers' markets.

As for poultry and eggs, the USDA organic certification described for meat and dairy applies in a similar way. However, other labels may be a little more ambiguous.

For example, "cage-free" means the animals do not live in cages but may still be confined in crowded indoor spaces with many other animals. "Free-range" means the animals have access to outdoor spaces, but the quality of that outdoor space and the amount of time they have to roam are not specified. "Pasture-raised," however, signifies that the animals have been raised outdoors. For example, pasture-raised chickens are generally able to eat grass and worms, which are their natural foods, and have more freedom to wander around. Your healthiest options are to look for organic or pasture-raised poultry and eggs.

A Whole World Under the Sea

Seafood has been touted as one of our healthiest sources of protein. However, because of our previous lack of awareness and urgency to mitigate our environmental impacts, we are no longer able to freely consume seafood. For example, because we have and still continue to pollute our waters every second of every day with our chemical-laden factories, agricultural practices, and municipal wastewater, many species of fish unavoidably ingest toxins their bodies cannot get rid of. When bigger fish prey on these little contaminated fish, the toxins are then passed up the food chain (called *bioaccumulation*). As a result, the higher-level predators within the food chain (i.e., swordfish, tuna, etc.) will end up with higher concentrations of pollutants inside their bodies as they eat hundreds or thousands of smaller, contaminated fish every day.

But this can happen to us as well! While the pollutants within any one fish are not nearly enough to kill us, we have yet to discover what bioaccumulation of toxins within *our* bodies can do to us over time.

Unfortunately, our past blind demands for specific types of fish, disregarding their conditions under the sea, have already led to over-exploitation of particular species. Many species of fish have become endangered or at risk of becoming endangered. As is discussed in the next chapter, the extinction of any one living species can cause detrimental chain reactions to its surrounding ecosystem. To prevent this, we need to avoid eating fish whose populations are already threatened and avoid purchasing ones caught using methods detrimental to the marine ecosystem.

Based on assessing the environmental impacts from various ways of fishing, the Natural Resources Defense Council (NRDC) recommends buying fish caught using the "hook and line" or "pots and traps" techniques while avoiding ones caught with "longlines" or "bottom trawlers,"[71] which are known to accidentally hurt and even kill other fish (known as "by-catch") not intended to be caught. Alternatively, you can head to Monterey Bay Aquarium's Seafood Watch website (SeafoodWatch.org) for their science-based, sustainable seafood shopping guide. There, the organization reveals the stories behind your fish, as well as potential concerns pertaining to each species. Finally, you can look out for sustainable seafood certifications, e.g., the Marine Stewardship Council certification, which denotes seafood caught or raised in more environmentally friendly ways.

Now that we know how impactful our food choices can be, it is in our hands to do things differently. If we want to be able to eat uncontaminated, healthy, diverse, nutritious food, we must collectively broaden our view of "healthy" and make more thoughtful consumer decisions.

Chapter Summary

Beauty From Within

Our foods are more than just foods. They each have a unique story of their own. Therefore, instead of judging them based solely on their physical properties, we need to seek beauty on a deeper level and shed light onto the **processes** behind their growth and production as well.

Revive Our Silent Springs

Since chemically toxic agricultural practices can pollute our air, water, and food, it matters what quality of produce you choose to buy. Whenever practical and possible, choose sustainably grown, nonsprayed produce over its conventional, chemical-laden counterparts.

Lower Yield; not a Big Deal

Our current food production is already more than enough to feed the entire world. Therefore, instead of attempting to maximize yield through toxic, chemical-intensive farming practices, we should aim to do so by improving the health of our lands. For sustainability, the quality of production is more important than the quantity.

The GMO Nondebate

Currently, with so many unknowns revolving around the widespread use of GMOs, there is not enough evidence for us to be completely pro- or anti-GMOs. So, for now, we should first support the sustainable food production methods already shown to work in harmony with nature (i.e., small-scale farming that minimizes the use of toxic chemicals, values biodiversity, and cares for our land).

Honor Our Farmers

In many cultures, the farmer's role is largely undermined and undervalued. Yet farmers are at the very forefront producing food vital to our health and taking care of lands vital to our planet's health. Thus, we must honor and respect our passionate and knowledgeable farmers and support agricultural practices that keep them financially secure, safe, healthy, and satisfied.

Chapter Summary (Cont'd)

Old MacDonald, Where's Your Farm?

Unfortunately, many of our animal farms today involve overpopulated cages, maltreated livestock, unnatural feed, and injections of antibiotics and hormones. However, for our meats and animal products to be healthy, the animals need to be healthy and happy first. So, for your welfare, the welfare of our animals, and our planet's overall welfare, choose high-quality animal products from livestock raised in humane, natural ways.

A Whole World Under the Sea

Due to our previous lack of urgency to mitigate our environmental impacts, many fish have become endangered or contaminated by our pollutants. To not exacerbate these problems any further through our everyday decisions, we must make more environmentally conscious choices, cut down on the amount of toxic or nonbiodegradable waste we generate, avoid eating fish at risk of becoming endangered, and avoid eating fish caught using methods harmful to the marine ecosystem.

Chapter 12

Nourish Our Lands

Whether you eat plants, plant-eating animals, or animal-eating carnivores, their nutrients can all be traced back to our lands (or aquatic environments for marine species). Therefore, for us to be healthy and for our food to be healthy, our lands must be healthy as well. To support a healthy planet that plants and animals can thrive on, we need to actively do two things:

1. mitigate our environmental impact, and

2. strengthen our efforts to conserve biodiversity.

I know—we often hear these things but feel that they are too grand for us to individually take on. In a way, they are. These overarching goals cannot be accomplished through any simple changes. Rather, they require changes from various approaches simultaneously. We must reshape our individual choices; businesses must use their powers for good; and organizations and governments must push for supporting policies and regulations.

But see—we *are* part of this picture, and we do have an integral part to play. So, have faith in your little day-to-day changes. I promise that you can make a positive difference simply by recrafting your own food choices.

Maintaining Biodiversity to Maintain Our Planet

To understand how we can best conserve biodiversity by our food choices, let us first examine the three levels of biodiversity: *genetic diversity, species diversity,* and *ecosystem diversity.*

Genetic Diversity

Genetic diversity refers to the variety of genes (what is passed down from parents to their offspring to determine the offspring's characteristics) among a species. Genetic diversity is crucial for maintaining the health of entire populations over time, because it allows the species to adapt to changes in the environment. Take, for example, a field of sunflowers. If every sunflower in that field contained the exact same genetic makeup that lacked resistance to droughts, all the sunflowers would be more likely to die when faced with a drought. On the other hand, if some sunflowers are resistant to droughts, some are able to tolerate floods, and some have better immune systems to protect against diseases, the field of sunflowers altogether is more likely to survive throughout time. As time goes on, the sunflowers that do survive any changes within the environment will then pass on their adaptability to their offspring, thus increasing the likelihood that their species will continue to thrive.

This is why we need to steer away from eating endangered animal or plant species, and why we cannot overexploit any one species. When any population size drops to alarming levels, their ability to adapt to changing environments will be threatened because of a decrease in gene variability.

Now, you might ask: "So what, if a species goes extinct?" To understand the answer to this question, we will need to examine the importance of species diversity.

Species Diversity

Species diversity refers to the variety of species within one *ecosystem* (an ecological community of living organisms and the components in their physical environment, like air and water). It takes into account both the number of different species present in a community (*species richness*) and the relative abundance of each species (*species evenness*).

For example, a field of 5 types of plants would be richer in species diversity than a field with just sunflowers. And a field of 10 sunflowers and 10 daisies would be more even in species diversity than a field of 1 sunflower and 19 daisies. Species richness helps to keep an ecosystem in balance, while species evenness minimizes the chances that any one species will die off by chance.

This level of biodiversity is crucial for an ecosystem's overall health, because every species in a community plays an integral role. Moreover, "even the loss of a few species from mature, diverse communities could lead in the long-term to decreases [in the sustainability of the ecosystem's functioning.]"[72]

Unfortunately, the extinction of any species can cause undesired chain reactions throughout an entire community. For example, bees are primary pollinators vital to many plants' survival. If all bees in a meadow were to disappear, the plants that depend on them would be wiped out next. In turn, other species that live off of the plants may die out, and so forth. Therefore, the endangerment of any one species signals more than just that; it represents a threat to an entire ecosystem's balance and health.

On farms, species diversity is key in helping to keep the soil naturally rich in nutrients. In fact, a study found that species-rich plots of land became richer in nitrogen (a nutrient vital to a plant's growth) over time, as compared to plots poorer in species diversity.[73] Although the health of our soil may seem irrelevant to us, the soil is actually where most of our nutrients originate from when we trace back each of our food chains. To ensure that our lands are lively and productive—so that our food will be nutritious—we will need to conserve biodiversity on our planet and *agrobiodiversity* (diversity of crops in agriculture) on our farms.

Of course, the value of species diversity is not limited to how it maintains an ecosystem's overall health. Do you ever find yourself fascinated by animals or plants you have never seen before? The truth is, biodiversity is also of economical value to us. For example, we often visit animal sanctuaries, stroll in botanical gardens or national parks, snorkel or scuba-dive at sea, or travel around the globe just to witness our world's natural wonders firsthand.

Moreover, the numerous species on our planet not only are direct sources of food for us but might also have potential medicinal values. Many of our drugs today are inspired by or derived from plant products. However, of the estimated 250,000 (to more than 750,000) plant species on earth, we have been using only around 90 species for medicine.[74] Perhaps the cure to cancer or other untreatable illnesses is already out there somewhere. But with every species that goes extinct, we also lose one more avenue of hope.

Ecosystem Diversity

Finally, *ecosystem diversity* refers to the different landscapes on our planet: deserts, tropical rain forests, tundras, wetlands, and so on. These various ecosystems are integral to our planet's overall balance and health, because they each have vital roles and functions.

For example, oceans stabilize the temperatures within our atmosphere, while forests are important *carbon sinks*, absorbing a lot of the carbon dioxide from our atmosphere, because plants absorb carbon dioxide, and tropical rain forests are extremely lush in vegetation.

Our world's wetlands—*half* of which were destroyed and converted into land fit for human use (i.e., agriculture or commercial development) since 1900 because in the past they were thought of as wastelands—are in fact among the most productive ecosystems in the world.[75] We must thus conserve our remaining wetlands, because these ecosystems help to attenuate the detrimental effects from extreme weather conditions such as hurricanes and also help to moderate climate change.

From the extremely dry to the extremely humid, from the extremely hot to the extremely cold, individual ecosystems may appear very different from one another. But their differences are what keep planet Earth balanced and healthy as a whole.

When we take a step back to examine the importance of the different levels of biodiversity, it becomes clear that we need:

- *genetic diversity,* to preserve healthy populations of individual species;

- *species diversity,* to maintain the health of independent ecosystems; and

- *ecosystem diversity,* to enhance the well-being of our planet as one whole.

Because we, as a species, are so impactful and have the ability to alter entire landscapes and even our global climate, it is our duty to become more mindful of our actions to ensure that we do not accidentally turn our powers against ourselves.

A Biodiverse Plate, a Biodiverse Planet

How has our food culture directly threatened biodiversity? The answer lies partly in the fact that we have altered our mindsets from an "eco-centric" view of food—understanding what our ecosystems can support and what our lands can grow in order to decide what we can eat—to a more "anthropocentric" view—asking ourselves what we want to eat in order to decide what and how much of it we need to grow. This has resulted in agricultural systems all over the world that do not mimic the way our complex ecosystems naturally function but only reflect our more simpleminded, profit-driven demand and supply.

According to the FAO, roughly 75% of plant genetic diversity within farms was lost between 1900 to 2000 as farmers abandoned their local crop varieties for genetically uniform ones.[76] What happened? Well, agriculture is a business, and farmers can earn money only from selling crops people buy. To meet the high demands of particular food types and to lessen their costs, many farmers adopted *monocropping* (i.e., only growing one species of crop on the farmland) to mass-produce and maximize the yield for one certain crop type. This increase in supply then led to lower purchase prices for consumers, making this monocropped produce even more appealing. However, monocropping makes a farm more vulnerable to pests and diseases, thus requiring more agrochemical use.

And, as we have discussed, our land cannot be naturally healthy without biodiversity.

While this is admittedly an oversimplified discussion of agrobiodiversity loss, the overall trend is clear. Decades of these vicious cycles later, our farms have lost dramatic amounts of species diversity, making our lands less healthy, and our diets have lost dramatic amounts of food diversity, making *us* less healthy. Now, 75% of the world's food is generated from only 12 plants and 5 animal species.[77] And of the tens of thousands of edible plant species known to us, we eat only 150 to 200 of them.[78]

However, there are so many more species of plants or types of animal products that may have important health-boosting properties for us. Our diets simply do not contain nearly as much variety as they should, and our farmlands are also not nearly as rich in biodiversity as they should be.

Of course, this is a bidirectional relationship. Without novel, local produce in our grocery stores, we have no choice but to choose what is available. This scenario proves that the conservation of local agrobiodiversity requires us to work together with our farmers.

If everyone wanted only potatoes, farmers might grow only potatoes, and significant areas of our planet would end up being covered in uniform potato fields. To help maintain agrobiodiversity, then, we need to diversify what we choose to put on our plates. Instead of going to the grocery store with a premade shopping list, try going empty-handed and see what novel, local varieties of vegetables and fruits you can find. Try not to buy the same types of produce two grocery trips in a row. Also, if a new type of produce is introduced at your local farmers' market, snatch it and get creative with it. When farmers begin reintroducing lesser-known, local crop varieties back into their farms, they will need our support to continue.

Plate Planet

When we compare the traditional diets of various populations, we see that all of their diets differ in their proportions of animal products, grains, vegetables, and fruits—depending on what was available to them in their environments. For example, populations that lived close to the ocean (such as the Japanese) thrived on mostly seafood, and populations that lived in the lush tropics thrived on a variety of animal and plant-based foods. Meanwhile, because the Arctic's Inuit populations and Tanzania and Kenya's Maasai populations lived in regions that lacked edible vegetation, meats and animal fats dominated their traditional diets.

Surprisingly, though, they had no more cardiovascular disease than other populations, likely due to the fact that their bodies had adapted to these diets and the animals they ate were healthy.[79,80]

What can we take away from all of this? First, as discussed in Chapter 9, "Sustain Your Body," remember that there is no perfect diet out there made for everyone. Through evolution, our bodies have adapted to thrive by eating whatever food was readily available in the regions we lived in. Therefore, instead of taking a strictly *anthropocentric* approach to eating (thinking only about what we *want* to eat), we can benefit by examining what diets our landscapes can actually support (adopting a more *eco-centric* approach). This way, we will be able to live more sustainably in harmony with our natural environments.

Second, all traditional diets involved *real foods*—namely, animal products from animals raised naturally or hunted from the wild, and plant-based foods grown within fertile, healthy soil. This suggests that we need to emphasize eating not just whole foods, but *quality* whole foods—ones grown or raised healthfully, as nature had intended them to be.

No matter what we each decide to eat, however, there is some universal truth to why we should collectively eat less meat and more plant-based foods. In terms of human health, almost all nutrition experts agree that many people do not eat enough fruits and vegetables, and that we would benefit by doing so. Many of us also overestimate our protein requirements and consume more protein than our bodies need in order to be healthy (see the "Remember the Purpose of Eating" section in Chapter 9). Instead of making animal-based, protein-rich foods the primary ingredient on our plates and having fiber-rich plant foods only as garnishes on the side, we can be just as healthy—if not healthier—by switching the two: having the plant foods as our main courses and the animal foods as our garnishes.

In terms of environmental health, we must remember the relationship our meals have to our planet's ecosystems. Because of how impactful we are to our planet, most of our plates need to reflect what is readily available in nature. Other than in regions of extreme climates where there may be a lack of edible vegetation, plants dominate most of our lands. Our planet simply cannot support everyone having carnivorous diets—especially ones rich in livestock-farmed beef, which is more energy, land, and water intensive compared to all other types of meat.[81-83] Therefore, eating in a sustainable manner to support the health of our planet requires the majority of us to adopt plant-based diets.

Maybe one day, when we collectively master the ability to think not only for our immediate health but also for our entire planet's long-term well-being, we will all be able to thrive together. That one day, our collective human diet will reflect what nature readily produces again, and our farms will become so rich in biodiversity that we may not even be able to tell them apart anymore from their surrounding, wild landscapes!

Chapter Summary

Maintaining Biodiversity to Maintain Our Planet

For our planet to be healthy, we need to preserve all three levels of biodiversity: **genetic diversity, species diversity,** and **ecosystem diversity**. As the endangerment of any one species signifies a threat to an entire ecosystem, we need to avoid overexploiting any one species and support efforts to conserve our planet's biodiversity.

A Biodiverse Plate, a Biodiverse Planet

To help preserve **agrobiodiversity** (biodiversity on our farms) to maintain the health of our farmlands, diversify what you choose to put on your plates. To help conserve the biodiversity in your region, try out local plants and vegetables you have never tried before, and support the comeback of any local, lesser-known crop varieties when they get introduced at your farmers' markets. Conveniently, incorporating more diversity into your diets will also improve your health.

Plate Planet

Because of how impactful we are as a species, most of what we eat must reflect what our natural ecosystems can support. Since plants dominate most of our lands, eating sustainably requires most of us to adopt plant-based diets. Plus, doing so will be advantageous for us, as the health benefits of eating more whole vegetables and fruits can be immediate and profound.

Chapter 13

Combine the Ingredients

Cooking, at its best, is an art form and a creative outlet. There is no right or wrong way to cook. This means cooking good food does not require us to strictly follow existing recipes. We have the freedom to decide what ingredients to use, where to get them, and how to cook or process them. When we combine this freedom we have as chefs with the connection our food has to our world as a whole, it becomes clear that cooking means much more than simply crafting dishes. Indeed, as the chef of your own kitchen, you can make choices that will help preserve your local landscape, support sustainable agriculture, reduce food waste, and enhance the health of your loved ones and your other diners. Doesn't that make you feel pretty powerful?

Cherish Local Landscapes

Why is Italian food so good in Italy and Japanese food so good in Japan? The cooking skills and experiences that have been passed down from generation to generation are sure factors, but I think the tasty seasonal and local ingredients readily available to them play an important role as well.

Throughout time, cuisines all over the world developed according to the food sources readily available within their regional environments and the imported crops that were able to thrive in their local climates. For example, Icelandic cuisine commonly involves seafood such as halibut, haddock, and plaice—species of fish commonly found in Iceland's surrounding North Atlantic Ocean. Mexican cuisine uses corn, a grain domesticated by the indigenous people of Mexico tens of thousands of years ago, as a staple food. And, Chinese cuisine often involves ingredients such as tofu from soybeans and vegetables such as *bok choy,* bean sprouts, and Chinese spinach. All of these typical Chinese vegetables have grown naturally in East Asian soil for hundreds and thousands of years. To truly understand food from various countries around the world requires us to examine the natural environments and climates they come from.

Fast forward to right now. In our supermarkets of today, you can find ingredients imported from all over the world and produce grown and harvested thousands of miles away. Unfortunately, because of the disconnect between us and our natural environments in our modern world, we are as far from understanding local and seasonal influences on the food we eat as we have ever been.

But there is hope. René Redzepi, executive chef and owner of Noma—a restaurant in Copenhagen, consistently ranked as one of the world's best—leads by example by bringing back a more eco-centric view of food. His philosophy of dining is the epitome of local and seasonal, as the chefs in his restaurant are asked to forage every day in the wild or on their farm to collect the freshest ingredients. Their menu changes every few weeks throughout the entire year, reflecting how the Scandinavian landscape evolves with the seasons. The result is a dining experience that is insightful, humbling, and down to earth—an experience that truly connects the diner with the Scandinavian natural environment.

To follow Redzepi's approach to sourcing ingredients and becoming a more purposeful, sustainability-oriented chef, we have to go from an anthropocentric view of cooking to a more eco-centric one. Instead of thinking, "I want to make an apple pie; let me acquire all the ingredients this apple pie recipe calls for," try to see first what ingredients are readily available this season within your local landscape.

Buying local and seasonal produce not only stimulates your local economy, but also reduces your so-called *food miles*, or the distance your food travels from its origin to you. On average, food within the United States travels a shocking distance of 1,500 miles (2,414 km) from origin to consumer.[84] Imagine how much energy you can help save and greenhouse gas emissions you can help reduce, simply by choosing local produce over imported produce! Since the level of nutrients within fruits and vegetables diminishes over time, eating freshly picked local produce can also maximize the amount of nutrients you get from your diet.

Especially at a time when we have lost touch with our natural environments, I truly believe that learning to understand our local landscapes to determine what to cook and eat can be a first step to reconnecting with nature. By shopping for a wide variety of seasonal, local, and responsibly grown produce for your recipes, your cooking will become more than just cooking. Instead of merely creating dishes, you will be crafting meaning. Instead of simply cooking because you need to eat, you will be cooking with a deeper purpose.

Trash-to-Table Cooking

For three weeks in March of 2015, world-renowned chef Dan Barber transformed Blue Hill, his restaurant in New York's Greenwich Village, into a concept pop-up restaurant, wastED. What was the concept? To "reconceive 'waste' that occurs at every link in the food chain."[85] Instead of crafting meals based solely on what would taste good, the chefs made gourmet dishes from ingredients typically tossed out as byproducts of the food system.

It's one thing to be able to combine any ingredient you want into delicious dishes, but it's quite another to be able to turn whatever you are given—even if that means food scraps—into gourmet meals. This made their chefs not only artists and masters in the kitchen, but also change-makers helping to address our global food-waste problems.

Although we may not all be master chefs, we ourselves can be change-making, waste-reducing cooks at home as well. Next time, before you decide what to make for dinner, first check your refrigerator to see what you already have on hand. Prioritize using up your perishable ingredients first, and then see what other groceries you may need to buy to complete the meal.

To address food waste, you can also implement the "root-to-stalk" and "nose-to-tail" principles. In "root-to-stalk" cooking, you use as much of the entire vegetable as possible from the roots to the leaves to the stems and stalk. For example, we typically only eat the florets of broccoli. However, there are many different ways you can turn its stalk into a dish, too. Different parts of a vegetable also contain different nutrients and phytonutrients. Therefore, cooking this way can also contribute to the variety in your diet. Before you try eating something novel, however, make sure the part is edible by searching for applicable recipes.

Similarly, "nose-to-tail" signifies that you eat not only the muscle-meat of animals, but also their livers, intestines, skin, tendons, etc. While you may cringe at the thought of eating any animal part other than the muscle-meat, all traditional diets have always included consuming animals in their entirety, not just picking out the muscle-meat. Plus, organ-meats such as the liver and kidneys are very dense in nutrition, often trumping the amount of nutrients found in muscle meat. For example, beef liver and kidneys are extremely rich in vitamin B_{12}, a micronutrient many people have deficiencies of. For equal grams of beef liver and beef tenderloin, beef liver contains 78 times more vitamin B_{12} than the muscle-meat! Therefore, eating a variety of quality animal parts not only reduces food waste, but also helps to maintain healthier nutritional profiles.

Water Your Plants, but Water Your Food, Too

From boiling to broiling, from simmering to searing, there are endless ways to turn our foods into scrumptious dishes. However, *cooking* is a way of "processing" food and altering its original chemistry, and certain ways of cooking can produce harmful substances such as AGEs (see Chapter 10). Thankfully, there are also cooking methods deemed healthier; most involve the various uses of moist heat, and are called "indirect" methods of cooking, where the source of heat (the flame) does not come in direct contact with the food being cooked. For optimum health, use these healthier methods of cooking as much as possible while minimizing the use of less healthy ones (see Table 13-1).

Table 13-1. Healthy Versus Less-Healthy Ways of Cooking

Healthy Ways of Cooking	Less-Healthy Ways of Cooking
Indirect-cooking methods: steaming, boiling, poaching, stewing, braising, simmering, en papillote, sous vide, baking, or other moist and indirect cooking methods	Direct-cooking methods: deep-frying, broiling, grilling, searing, burning, charring, or any other dry and high temperature cooking methods
Tips: Try not to burn or char your food, especially your meats! Instead, cook at low to medium temperatures, add moisture to your cooking, or add acidic marinades such as lemon juice or vinegar.	

Nutritionally speaking, there are benefits to keeping your plant-based foods raw, like in salads, but also benefits in cooking them. As Registered Dietitian and culinary educator Kayleen St. John noted, some nutrients are lost or destroyed by the cooking process (i.e., vitamins B and C), but others are enhanced from exposure to heat (i.e., minerals).[86] So eat a *variety* of whole foods prepared in a *variety* of healthy methods. Embrace both your mixed salads and your Italian minestrone soups!

Ready, Reset, Go!

By now, I hope you have begun to see the true meaning behind your everyday food choices and understand how your diet connects you to our planet's ecosystem as a whole. As discussed in Part I, "Smile," some key elements of a fulfilling life include being able to find meaning in what you do and developing a connection to something larger than yourself. Although these tasks may sound complex, abstract, or even impossible, you can accomplish them both by simply re-shaping your perspective on food.

It might take some time for you to adjust to your new, healthier eating habits and decisions. However, the so-called bland taste from focusing on less-processed and more wholesome foods will soon start to change into a more delicious sensation than ever as you reset your palate, and it becomes more sensitive to even mild, subtle flavors. You will start to pick up more on the natural sweetness of cooked vegetables and the natural aromas of herbs and spices. You will begin to savor the real flavors of your dishes and open your senses to many, many more flavors beyond the typical sweet and salty.

Instead of seeing food as magically appearing in grocery stores, restaurants, or at your dining table, think about what your food really represents. The tastes and aromas of your meals may make eating enjoyable, but being able to build context around your food makes your dining experience so much more meaningful. Beyond your five senses, you can choose to engage your mind and heart in the experience and journey. By digging deeper to understand your food's roots, you may begin to see how much power you have as a chef or diner and how many opportunities lie before you every day to better your health and the health of our planet. As *Omnivore's Dilemma* author Michael Pollan noted, "The wonderful thing about food is you get three votes a day. Every one of them has the potential to change the world."

Chapter Summary

Cherish Local Landscapes

To cook sustainably, we will need to shift our perspective of food from an **anthropocentric** one to an **eco-centric** one. In other words, try to look at what is available in your regional landscape to determine what ingredients to buy or create dishes with.

Trash-to-Table Cooking

To cook sustainably, we also need to cut down on the amount of food waste we generate. When cooking at home, prioritize using up ingredients with quickly approaching expiration dates first, and then shop for additional groceries to complete the meal. Additionally, try to implement the **"root-to-stalk"** (eating as much of an entire vegetable as possible) and **"nose-to-tail"** (eating as many different parts of an animal as possible) concepts of eating when you make your food choices.

Water Your Plants, but Water Your Food, Too

Water is your best friend in cooking. For optimal health, cook as much as possible using **moist heat**, lower temperatures, and acidic ingredients. Meanwhile, cook less often with high temperatures and dry heat (which will more likely lead to the production of harmful substances such as AGEs in your food).

Ready, Reset, Go!

Yes, altering your eating habits and way of looking at food will take time to get used to. However, being able to judge your food from not only its physical properties, but also its rich history, can help make your dining experience more meaningful and your diet more sustainable!

Part References

1　Damasceno, A., & Steyn, K. (2006). Lifestyle and related risk factors for chronic diseases. In K. Steyn (Author), *Disease and mortality in Sub-Saharan Africa*. Washington, D.C.: World Bank

2　World Health Organization. (2006). *Constitution of the World Health Organization*. Retrieved from http://www.who.int/governance/eb/who_constitution_en.pdf

3　Minger, D. (2014). *Death by food pyramid: How shoddy science, sketchy politics and shady special interests have conspired to ruin the health of America* (1st ed.). Malibu, CA: Primal Blueprint Publishing.

4　Hu, F. B. (2010). Are refined carbohydrates worse than saturated fat? *American Journal of Clinical Nutrition, 91*(6), 1541-1542.

5　Lichtenstein, A. H., Kennedy, E., Barrier, P., Danford, D., Ernst, N. D., Grundy, S. M., . . . Booth, S. L. (1998). Dietary fat consumption and health. *Nutrition Reviews, 56*(5), 3-19.

6　Hoenselaar, R. (2012). Saturated fat and cardiovascular disease: The discrepancy between the scientific literature and dietary advice. *Nutrition, 28*(2), 118-123.

7　Hu, F. B. (2010). Are refined carbohydrates worse than saturated fat? *American Journal of Clinical Nutrition, 91*(6), 1541-1542.

8　Siri-Tarino, P. W., Sun, Q., Hu, F. B., & Krauss, R. M. (2010). Meta-analysis of prospective cohort studies evaluating the association of saturated fat with cardiovascular disease. *American Journal of Clinical Nutrition, 91*(3), 535-546.

9　Smit, L. A., Baylin, A., & Campos, H. (2010). Conjugated linoleic acid in adipose tissue and risk of myocardial infarction. *American Journal of Clinical Nutrition, 92*(1), 34-40.

10　Holmberg, S., & Thelin, A. (2013). High dairy fat intake related to less central obesity: A male cohort study with 12 years' follow-up. *Scandinavian Journal of Primary Health Care, 31*(2), 89-94.

11　Kratz, M., Baars, T., & Guyenet, S. (2013). The relationship between high-fat dairy consumption and obesity, cardiovascular, and metabolic disease. *European Journal of Nutrition, 52*(1), 1-24.

12　Natural Gourmet Institute. (2016, February). *Culinary nutrition*. Lecture presented at Natural Gourmet Institute, Los Angeles.

13   University of Illinois. (2004, February 4). *Macronutrients: The importance of carbohydrate, protein, and fat.* Retrieved from http://www.mckinley.illinois.edu/handouts/macronutrients.htm

14   United States Department of Agriculture. (2015). *Choose MyPlate.* Retrieved from http://www.choosemyplate.gov/about

15   United States Department of Agriculture. (2015). *Choose MyPlate.* Retrieved from http://www.choosemyplate.gov/about

16   Guallar, E., Stranges, S., Mulrow, C., Appel, L. J., & Miller, E. R. (2013). Enough is enough: Stop wasting money on vitamin and mineral supplements. *Annals of Internal Medicine, 159*(12), 850-851.

17   Sense About Science. (2009). *Debunking detox.* Retrieved from http://www.senseaboutscience.org/pages/debunking-detox.html

18   British Nutrition Foundation. (2013). *Understanding satiety: Feeling full after a meal.* Retrieved from http://www.nutrition.org.uk/healthyliving/fuller/understanding-satiety-feeling-full-after-a-meal.html

19   Heilbronn, L., & Ravussin, E. (2003). Calorie restriction and aging: Review of the literature and implications for studies in humans. *The American Journal of Clinical Nutrition, 27*(3), 361-369.

20   Heilbronn, L., & Ravussin, E. (2003). Calorie restriction and aging: Review of the literature and implications for studies in humans. *The American Journal of Clinical Nutrition, 27*(3), 361-369.

21   Bales, C. W., & Kraus, W. E. (2013). Caloric restriction. *Journal of Cardiopulmonary Rehabilitation and Prevention, 33*(4), 201-208.

22   Heilbronn, L., & Ravussin, E. (2003). Calorie restriction and aging: Review of the literature and implications for studies in humans. *The American Journal of Clinical Nutrition, 27*(3), 361-369.

23   American Heart Association. (2013). *Skipping breakfast may increase coronary heart disease risk.* Retrieved from http://newsroom.heart.org/news/skipping-breakfast-may-increase-coronary-heart-disease-risk

24   Adolphus, K., Lawton, C. L., & Dye, L. (2013). The effects of breakfast on behavior and academic performance in children and adolescents. *Frontiers in Human Neuroscience, 7,* 425.

25   Damasceno, A., & Steyn, K. (2006). Lifestyle and related risk factors for chronic diseases. In K. Steyn (Author), *Disease and mortality in Sub-Saharan Africa.* Washington, D.C.: World Bank.

26 Drewnowski, A., & Almiron-Roig, E. (2009). Human perceptions and preferences for fat-rich foods: Taste, texture, and post-ingestive effects. *Frontiers in Neuroscience Fat Detection*, 265-291.

27 Hu, F. B. (2010). Are refined carbohydrates worse than saturated fat? *American Journal of Clinical Nutrition*, *91*(6), 1541-1542.

28 Johnson, R. K., Appel, L. J., Brands, M., Howard, B. V., Lefevre, M., Lustig, R. H., . . . Wylie-Rosett, J. (2009). Dietary sugars intake and cardiovascular health: A scientific statement from the American Heart Association. *Circulation*, *120*(11), 1011-1020.

29 Liu, S., Willett, W., Stampfer, M., Hu, F., Franz, M., Sampson, L., . . . Manson, J. (2000). A prospective study of dietary glycemic load, carbohydrate intake, and risk of coronary heart disease in US women. *The American Journal of Clinical Nutrition*, *71*(6), 1455-1461.

30 Uribarri, J., Woodruff, S., Goodman, S., Cai, W., Chen, X., Pyzik, R., . . . Vlassara, H. (2010). Advanced glycation end products in foods and a practical guide to their reduction in the diet. *Journal of the American Dietetic Association*, *110*(6), 911-916.

31 Favell, D. (1998). A comparison of the vitamin C content of fresh and frozen vegetables. *Food Chemistry*, *62*(1), 59-64.

32 Hunter, K. J., & Fletcher, J. M. (2002). The antioxidant activity and composition of fresh, frozen, jarred and canned vegetables. *Innovative Food Science & Emerging Technologies*, *3*(4), 399-406.

33 Natural Gourmet Institute. (2016, February). *Culinary nutrition*. Lecture presented at Natural Gourmet Institute, Los Angeles.

34 Cook, J. D., & Reddy, M. B. (2001). Effect of ascorbic acid intake on non-heme-iron absorption from a complete diet. *The American Journal of Clinical Nutrition*, *73*(1), 93-98.

35 Hallberg, L., Brune, M., & Rossander, L. (1989). The role of vitamin C in iron absorption. *International Journal for Vitamin and Nutrition Research*, *30*, 103-108.

36 Butt, M. S., Pasha, I., Sultan, M. T., Randhawa, M. A., Saeed, F., & Ahmed, W. (2013). Black pepper and health claims: A comprehensive treatise. *Critical Reviews in Food Science and Nutrition*, *53*(9), 875-886.

37 Meghwal, M., & Goswami, T. K. (2013). Piper nigrum and Piperine: An update. *Phytotherapy Research*, *27*(8), 1121-1130.

38 Veda, S., & Srinivasan, K. (2009). Influence of dietary spices—Black pepper, red pepper and ginger on the uptake of β-carotene by rat intestines. *Journal of Functional Foods*, *1*(4), 394-398.

39 Muraki, I., Imamura, F., Manson, J. E., Hu, F. B., Willett, W. C., Dam, R. M., & Sun, Q. (2013). Fruit consumption and risk of type 2 diabetes: Results from three prospective longitudinal cohort studies. *British Medical Journal, 347*, f5001.

40 Bazzano, L. A., Li, T. Y., Joshipura, K. J., & Hu, F. B. (2008). Intake of fruit, vegetables, and fruit juices and risk of diabetes in women. *Diabetes Care, 31*(7), 1311-1317.

41 Muraki, I., Imamura, F., Manson, J. E., Hu, F. B., Willett, W. C., Dam, R. M., & Sun, Q. (2013). Fruit consumption and risk of type 2 diabetes: Results from three prospective longitudinal cohort studies. *British Medical Journal, 347*, f5001.

42 National Institute on Alcohol Abuse and Alcoholism. (n.d.). *Drinking levels defined.* Retrieved from http://www.niaaa.nih.gov/alcohol-health/overview-alcohol-consumption/moderate-binge-drinking

43 Naughton, D. P., & Petróczi, A. (2008). Heavy metal ions in wines: Meta-analysis of target hazard quotients reveal health risks. *Chemistry Central Journal, 2*(1), 22.

44 United States Department of Agriculture. (2010). *Dietary guidelines for Americans.* Retrieved from http://health.gov/dietaryguidelines/2010/

45 Curl, C. L., Beresford, S. A., Fenske, R. A., Fitzpatrick, A. L., Lu, C., Nettleton, J. A., & Kaufman, J. D. (2015). Estimating pesticide exposure from dietary intake and organic food choices: The multi-ethnic study of atherosclerosis (MESA). *Environmental Health Perspectives, 123*(5), 475-483.

46 Lu, C., Toepel, K., Irish, R., Fenske, R. A., Barr, D. B., & Bravo, R. (2006). Organic diets significantly lower children's dietary exposure to organophosphorus pesticides. *Environmental Health Perspectives, 114*(2), 260-263.

47 Leiss, J. K., & Savitz, D. A. (1995). Home pesticide use and childhood cancer: A case-control study. *American Journal of Public Health, 85*(2), 249-252.

48 Lucio, G. C. (2008). Neurotoxicity of pesticides: A brief review. *Frontiers in Bioscience, 13*(13), 1240.

49 Natural Resources Defense Council. (2012). *Pesticides: What you need to know.* Retrieved from http://www.nrdc.org/health/pesticides/

50 Shim, Y. K., Mlynarek, S. P., & Wijngaarden, E. V. (2009). Parental exposure to pesticides and childhood brain cancer: US Atlantic Coast childhood brain cancer study. *Environmental Health Perspectives, 117*(6), 1002-1006.

51 Zahm, S. H., & Ward, M. H. (1998). Pesticides and childhood cancer. *Environmental Health Perspectives, 106*, 893.

52   Clement, B. R. (2012). *Food is medicine.* Summertown, TN: Hippocrates Publications.

53   Food and Agriculture Organization of the United Nations. (2013). *Food waste foodprint: Impacts on natural resources* (Rep.). Retrieved from http://www.fao.org/docrep/018/i3347e/i3347e.pdf

54   Stuart, T. (2009). *Waste: Uncovering the global food scandal.* New York: W.W. Norton & Company, p xx.

55   Stuart, T. (2009). *Waste: Uncovering the global food scandal.* New York: W.W. Norton & Company, p 82.

56   Institute of Medicine, & National Research Council. (2004). *Safety of genetically engineered foods: Approaches to assessing unintended health effects.* Washington, DC: National Academies Press.

57   Kishi, M., Hirschhorn, N., Djajadisastra, M., Satterlee, L., Strowman, S., & Dilts, R. (1995). Relationship of pesticide spraying to signs and symptoms in Indonesian farmers. *Scandinavian Journal of Work, Environment & Health, 21*(2), 124-133.

58   Fleming, L. E., Gómez-MariN, O., Zheng, D., Ma, F., & Lee, D. (2003). National Health interview survey of mortality among US farmers and pesticide applicators. *American Journal of Industrial Medicine, 43*(2), 227-233.

59   Behere, P., & Bhise, M. (2009). Farmers' suicide: Across culture. *Indian Journal of Psychiatry, 51*(4), 242.

60   Fraser, C. E., Smith, K. B., Judd, F., Humphreys, J. S., Fragar, L. J., & Henderson, A. (2005). Farming and mental health problems and mental illness. *International Journal of Social Psychiatry, 51*(4), 340-349.

61   McCurdy, S. A., & Carroll, D. J. (2000). Agricultural injury. *American Journey of Industrial Medicine, 38*(4), 463-480.

62   Behere, P., & Bhise, M. (2009). Farmers' suicide: Across culture. *Indian Journal of Psychiatry, 51*(4), 242.

63   Gliessman, S. R., & Rosemeyer, M. (2010). *The conversion to sustainable agriculture: Principles, processes, and practices.* Boca Raton, FL: CRC Press.

64   Mzoughi, N. (2014). Do organic farmers feel happier than conventional ones? An exploratory analysis. *Ecological Economics, 103*, 38-43.

65   Steinfield, H., Gerber, P., Wassenaar, T., Castel, V., Rosales, M., & Haan, C. (2006). *Livestock's long shadow: Environmental issues and options* (Rep.). Rome: United Nations Food and Agriculture Organization. Retrieved from ftp://ftp.fao.org/docrep/fao/010/a0701e/a0701e00.pdf

66 Andersen, A. & Khun, K. (Directors). (2014). Cowspiracy [Motion picture documentary].

67 Aurousseau, B., Bauchart, D., Calichon, E., Micol, D., & Priolo, A. (2004). Effect of grass or concentrate feeding systems and rate of growth on triglyceride and phospholipid and their fatty acids in the M. longissimus thoracis of lambs. *Meat Science, 66*(3), 531-541.

68 Daley, C. A., Abbott, A., Doyle, P. S., Nader, G. A., & Larson, S. (2010). A review of fatty acid profiles and antioxidant content in grass-fed and grain-fed beef. *Nutrition Journal, 9*(1), 10.

69 Smit, L. A., Baylin, A., & Campos, H. (2010). Conjugated linoleic acid in adipose tissue and risk of myocardial infarction. *American Journal of Clinical Nutrition, 92*(1), 34-40.

70 Daley, C. A., Abbott, A., Doyle, P. S., Nader, G. A., & Larson, S. (2010). A review of fatty acid profiles and antioxidant content in grass-fed and grain-fed beef. *Nutrition Journal, 9*(1), 10.

71 Natural Resources Defense Council. (2014). *Sustainable seafood guide.* Retrieved from http://www.nrdc.org/oceans/seafoodguide/default.asp

72 Reich, P. B., Tilman, D., Isbell, F., Mueller, K., Hobbie, S. E., Flynn, D. F., & Eisenhauer, N. (2012). Impacts of biodiversity loss escalate through time as redundancy fades. *Science, 336*(6081), 589-592.

73 Reich, P. B., Tilman, D., Isbell, F., Mueller, K., Hobbie, S. E., Flynn, D. F., & Eisenhauer, N. (2012). Impacts of biodiversity loss escalate through time as redundancy fades. *Science, 336*(6081), 589-592.

74 Farnsworth, N. R. (1988). Screening plants for new medicines. In F. M. Peter & E. O. Wilson (Authors), *Biodiversity* (pp. 83-96). Washington, D.C.: National Academy Press.

75 Verhoeven, J. T., & Setter, T. L. (2009). Agricultural use of wetlands: Opportunities and limitations. *Annals of Botany, 105*(1), 155-163.

76 Food and Agriculture Organization of the United Nations. (2004). *What is agrobiodiversity?* (Rep.). Retrieved from ftp://ftp.fao.org/docrep/fao/007/y5609e/y5609e00.pdf

77 Food and Agriculture Organization of the United Nations. (2004). *What is agrobiodiversity?* (Rep.). Retrieved from ftp://ftp.fao.org/docrep/fao/007/y5609e/y5609e00.pdf

78 Food and Agriculture Organization of the United Nations. (2004). *What is agrobiodiversity?* (Rep.). Retrieved from ftp://ftp.fao.org/docrep/fao/007/y5609e/y5609e00.pdf

79 Dewailly, E., Blanchet, C., Lemieux, S., Sauvé, L., Gingras, S., Ayotte, P., & Holub, B. (2001). N−3 Fatty acids and cardiovascular disease risk factors among the Inuit of Nunavik. *The American Journal of Clinical Nutrition, 74*(4), 464-473.

80 Mann, G., Shaffer, R., Anderson, R., Sandstead, H., Prendergast, H., Mann, J., . . . Dicks, K. (1964). Cardiovascular disease in the Masai. *Journal of Atherosclerosis Research, 4*(4), 289-312.

81 Pimentel, D., & Pimentel, M. (2003). Sustainability of meat-based and plant-based diets and the environment. *The American Journal of Clinical Nutrition, 78*(3).

82 Weber, C. L., & Matthews, H. S. (2008). Food-miles and the relative climate impacts of food choices in the United States. *Environmental Science & Technology, 42*(10), 3508-3513.

83 White, T. (2000). Diet and the distribution of environmental impact. *Ecological Economics, 34*(1), 145-153.

84 DeWeerdt, S. (2009). Is local food better? *World Watch Magazine, 22*(3). Retrieved from http://www.worldwatch.org/

85 wastED (2016). About wastED. Retrieved from http://www.wastedny.com/

86 Natural Gourmet Institute. (2016, February). *Culinary nutrition.* Lecture presented at Natural Gourmet Institute, Los Angeles.

PART IV

BEAUTIFY

*"People often say that beauty is in the eye of the beholder,
and I say that the most liberating thing about beauty is realizing you are
the beholder."*
—Salma Hayek

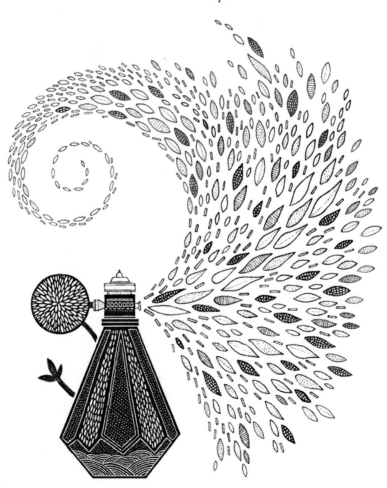

Chapter 14

Choose Safety First

That new, citrus-scented body spray? Chances are, you are not smelling real lemons, but just a chemical concoction that may contain neurotoxins.

Your new exfoliator? It may contain plastic microbeads that can end up sitting in lakes for centuries, or even end up inside your fish for dinner.

If you think all of the ingredients in your shampoos and self-care products have been tested and proven to be safe and healthy, I must sadly tell you that you are wrong. Ironically, the products you have been using to maintain and enhance your appearance may be slowly deteriorating your health.

Body Pollution

Under the United States 1938 Food, Drugs, and Cosmetics Act, only drugs must go through rigorous testing before they can be put onto the market. Meanwhile, the safety of self-care products has been left entirely up to the companies for "self-regulation" because these products were made for only cleansing, promoting attractiveness, or altering appearances on the surface of one's skin.

However, when the law was enacted, skin was usually thought of as an impermeable, dead tissue. We now know that this is completely false. Skin is actually our human body's largest organ and serves many important functions, such as protection against harmful microbes, tactile sensation, excretion of waste products, vitamin D synthesis, and temperature regulation.[1] Unfortunately, no reforms have been made to that law, and ingredients that are potentially harmful to us or to our planet can still be used in our self-care products.

What may be even more alarming is that most chemicals on the market—which amount to more than 80,000—have never been tested.[2] Scientists from the President's Cancer Panel even said that babies today are born "pre-polluted," as the scientists have discovered numerous contaminants that are able to cross the placental barrier, an organ that regulates the exchange of substances between a mother and her growing fetus during pregnancy.[3] Considering that the average American woman uses 12 products a day, including 168 unique ingredients, while the average American man uses 6 products a day with 85 unique ingredients, we need to become educated consumers so we will not accidentally harm ourselves in the name of beauty.[4]

Justified Concerns

For the most part, our skin does an amazing job at keeping toxins out of our bodies. While our skin certainly does not drink up everything we put on it, however, it is capable of absorbing substances it comes in contact with, depending on various factors, including:

- *skin integrity,* or the condition the skin is in (i.e., intact or damaged);
- where on our bodies our skin is exposed;
- the physical and chemical properties of the substances used;
- the concentration of the substance on your skin;
- the duration of exposure; and
- the surface area, or how much of your body is exposed.[5]

A recent study found that urinary metabolites of triphenyl phosphate—a plasticizer often used in nail polish that may disrupt hormone balance and affect the liver and kidneys—increased seven times following the application of nail polish.[6, 7] Another study examining mineral oil hydrocarbons, one of the greatest contaminants of the human body, concluded that cosmetic products could be important and relevant sources.[8] Finally, adverse skin reactions from cosmetic products most commonly come from those that remain *on* the skin, such as moisturizers, lotions, tonics, nail varnish, hair dyes, perfumes, and makeup products.[9]

All of these findings confirm that our skin is *alive* and constantly interacts with the substances it comes in contact with. Given the industry's current lack of stringent regulations, we must start asking questions, establishing our priorities, and finding healthier cosmetic products for ourselves.

At the current moment, low concentrations of chemicals suspected or shown to have harmful effects on animals or humans are still allowed in our consumer products. While the amounts of these chemicals in individual products are unlikely to hurt us directly and immediately, there are more parts to the equation that we need to think about.

As mentioned above, because of the interactive relationship between our health and the health of our planet, we need to broaden our definition of "healthy." To label a product as truly healthy or safe, then, we need to consider both its direct and indirect effects. This means the potential impacts from a product's *entire lifecycle*—including the ingredient sourcing, production, transport, use, and disposal phases—need to be considered. We also need to not only consider a product's potential health risks to the end consumer, but also:

- Potential health risks to people exposed regularly to larger quantities of the product (e.g. cosmetologists, people who work in cosmetics manufacturers, etc.), the chemicals in them, as well as the byproducts from manufacturing;

- Potential health risks to our planet's ecosystem (biodegradability of the product and its packaging; toxicity to wildlife; potential to pollute our lands, waterways, and air, etc.).

Preventative Care

By definition, every chemical, whether natural or synthetic, can be "toxic," depending on the dosage.[10] Even water can be toxic if consumed in a large amount in a short period of time! However, using this idea to justify the safe use of *low doses* of chemicals shown or suspected to have detrimental effects on our bodies (carcinogens, neurotoxins, hormone disruptors, etc.) in our daily products undermines the complexity of toxicology.

First, long-term exposures to low doses of certain chemicals can have cumulative effects and lead to chronic illnesses.[11] According to the NRDC, "There is growing recognition in the scientific community that exposure to even low doses of certain chemicals, particularly in the womb or during early childhood, can disturb our hormonal, reproductive, and immune systems, and that multiple chemicals can act together to harm human health."[12] On top of this, some chemicals can be toxic no matter what their dosage, and everyone's body differs in how sensitive it is to different substances.

As you can see, all of these variables make it extremely challenging to comprehensively determine a chemical's short-term and long-term effects. However, rather than gamble with our health on these uncertainties, we can use the Precautionary Principle to practice preventative care; that is, we can reduce the possibilities of potential harm by minimizing our exposures to chemicals shown or even suspected to have any detrimental effects at all.

Chapter Summary

Body Pollution

Currently, ingredients suspected or shown to be harmful to humans, animals, or our ecosystem are still allowed in our cosmetic products at varying concentrations. Since most commercially used chemicals have never been tested, we each use multiple products every day, and chemical pollution is becoming a worldwide problem, we need to become educated consumers so we do not accidentally hurt our health or the health of our environment in the name of beauty.

Justified Concerns

Since our skin is capable of absorbing substances it comes in contact with (depending on various factors), what we choose to put on our skin can affect our health. Moreover, because our well-being depends on the health of our planet as a whole, we need to apply our broadened definition of 'healthy' to our cosmetics products, too. Instead of only considering whether a product is safe for us to use for the short-term, we also need to consider its long-term impacts to our ecosystem and to the people who are exposed regularly to larger quantities of the product (cosmetologists, factory workers, etc.).

Preventative Care

Instead of gambling with our health on all of the unknowns from our under-regulated cosmetics industry, we can take a more **preventative approach** by minimizing the purchase of products containing ingredients established, or even suspected, to be harmful to human or environmental health.

Chapter 15

Shop Mindfully

Did you know that many of the shampoos sold commercially contain *sodium lauryl sulfate*, a known skin irritant that may contribute to hair loss? Or that the inhalation of *toluene*—an ingredient often used in nail polish—by pregnant women has been associated with *feto-toxicity* (toxicity to fetuses), retardation of the fetus within the uterus, premature delivery, congenital malformations, and postnatal developmental retardation?[14]

It's not that anyone is trying to hurt us—but simply that when these chemicals were first used, their health effects were not fully understood. Unfortunately, as the number of commercially used chemicals (whose effects we don't fully understand) continues to rise, our health risks only rise with it. Clearly, something needs to change.

Questionable Until Proven Safe

Last summer, when I travelled through Scandinavia, I fell in love with water. I watched it ripple elegantly in the Norwegian fjords, and I watched it gush powerfully down grand waterfalls in Iceland. In Voss, I drank the purest and most refreshing water I had ever tasted in my life—straight out of the waterfall streams. Suddenly, water became more than just water to me. Witnessing its natural flow in the wilderness made me realize it had a beautiful story of its own—a story that needed to be remembered and appreciated, yet a story often undervalued. Wouldn't it be wonderful if we could drink purified water—naturally enriched with minerals from our lands—without the need to worry about potential chemical pollutants? Unfortunately, we are only drifting further away from that possibility.

Alarmingly, 44% of tested stream miles and 64% of tested lake acres within the United States are considered "impaired," meaning unsafe for any water activities.[15] This means no swimming, no fishing, and definitely no drinking.

How did this happen? Once again, the "innocent until proven dangerous" approach to regulating chemicals is to blame. According to the Environmental Working Group, more than 200 unregulated chemicals have been found in the tap water of 45 states.[16] If the potential negative side effects of new chemicals are not yet well understood, they will not be regulated. And if they are not regulated, they are allowed to be in our drinking water—no matter how high their concentrations. Of course, the chemicals polluting our waterways come from not only our municipal wastewater—which is contaminated by everything we wash down the drain—but also agricultural wastes and agrochemicals, effluent from factories and manufacturing plants, oil-drilling, corrosion of old pipelines, and so on.

To make matters worse, even *regulated* chemicals can end up in our drinking water. In April 2014, a water contamination crisis in Flint, Michigan, emerged. When the city switched their water source from Detroit Water and Sewerage Department water to the Flint River to cut costs, it failed to comprehensively test and treat its new water supply. Unfortunately, Flint's new drinking water was contaminated with dangerously high levels of lead, and tens of thousands of citizens—including thousands of children—have been exposed ever since. This resulted in the Governor of Michigan and President Obama declaring the city to be in a public health state of emergency—but only more than a year later.

While this water contamination resulted primarily from the corrosion of old pipelines (rather than from factory effluent, agricultural runoff, or our wastewater), it still illustrates two very important points:

1. We cannot be absolutely certain that water deemed "safe to drink" is free of all unregulated—or even regulated—toxic chemicals.

2. Without a more preventative approach to keeping our environment clean, we will always be one step behind.

Even if certain chemicals may be harmless to humans, their use should still be minimized if they pose any threat to other animals or the environment, or if they are not biodegradable. According to the International Joint Commission, only about half of the newly emerging contaminants in sewages are actually filtered out by treatment plants.[17] Because our current wastewater systems cannot remove all of the increasing numbers of chemicals that contaminate our water, these chemicals may end up bypassing our wastewater treatments and polluting our water sources. Unfortunately, "When streams become overloaded with pollution or nonbiodegradable man-made ingredients (contaminants), the stream's natural purification processes cannot return the water to its normal quality."[18]

So what can we do? In the grander scheme of things, we will need to push for a system of regulation that focuses on *problem prevention*, not potential problem creation. This "innocent until proven dangerous" approach to regulating chemicals will simply not suffice. By the time a chemical proves itself to be harmful, it may already have caused irreversible damage. Since clean water, clean air, and diverse, nutritious foods are our only physical necessities to good health, we must ask: Why are we allowing ourselves to be the guinea pigs in a giant, uncontrolled, unconsented experiment?

Although we cannot stop all forms of pollution through our consumer choices, we can still play an important part by establishing our priorities and turning our everyday purchases into meaningful statements.

Better Safe Than Sorry

Finding healthy, eco-conscious self-care products will take a little effort when you begin to search for them. However, once you get the hang of what to look out for, it will only get easier. Since product descriptions on the label, such as "natural" or even "dermatologist tested," are unregulated, looking for the more factual information, such as the list of ingredients, is a much more reliable indicator of the product's potential effects.

In Table 15-1 on the next page, you will find a qualitative reference that will help you pick out some of the most common cosmetic ingredients that are:

- Known or probable *carcinogens* (cause cancer), *endocrine disruptors* (disrupt hormones), *mutagenic ingredients* (mutate cells), and other substances harmful to body cells;

- Known skin irritants and common *allergens* (cause allergies);

- Likely to be contaminated with or produce harmful byproducts; or

- *Nonbiodegradable* (will not readily break down in nature) environmental pollutants or ingredients that can threaten environmental health.

Keep in mind that this guide is but a snapshot of what potentially harmful ingredients you may be exposed to on a regular basis within your self-care products. (See also Table 15-2, which categorizes the ingredients according to what products typically carry them.) It is by no means exhaustive, as the number of commercially used chemicals continues to increase, and our understanding of these chemicals continues to improve. Therefore, I highly encourage you to learn more on your own to make your own set of informed decisions.

Table 15-1. Beware of These Ingredients[19-23]

Ingredient	What's the catch?
1,4 dioxane	• Probable human carcinogen • Capable of penetrating animal and human skin • Not typically used as an ingredient, but according to the Environmental Working Group (2008), contaminates up to 46% of personal care products tested • Likely to contaminate otherwise safe petroleum-based ingredients, such as "PEG," "polyethylene," "polyethylene glycol," "polyoxyethylene," etc.
Benzene	• Known human carcinogen
Coal tar	• Byproduct of coal processing • Known human carcinogen
Dibutyl Phthalate (DBP)	• May be a teratogen (mutate the embryo) • May damage developing fetus and testes • May affect nervous system and kidneys
DMDM Hydantoin	• May release formaldehyde (see formaldehyde)
Formaldehyde	• Know human carcinogen • Ingredients that may release formaldehyde: DMDM hydantoin, diazolidinyl urea, imidzaolidinyl urea, and quaternium-15
Fragrance	• Meaningless when listed as an ingredient • Easily inhaled, and the chemicals within may enter bloodstreams • May contain harmful ingredients • One of the most common allergens • "Unscented" can still be an odor-masking fragrance
Hydroquinone	• Carcinogenicity demonstrated in animals • Unclassified carcinogenicity in humans • Skin irritant • Occupational chronic exposure may lead to adverse health effects
Lead	• Neurotoxin, especially in infants and toddlers • Probable carcinogen
Loose powders/ aerosol spray	• Easily inhaled, which may then be absorbed into the bloodstream from the lungs • Some ingredients are safe topically, but not when inhaled • If possible, choose cream products instead

Table 15-1. Beware of These Ingredients Cont'd

Ingredient	What's the catch?
Methylene chloride	• Carcinogenic to animals • Often found in hair spray • Chronic exposure may damage central nervous system
Mineral oil	• Mildly treated mineral oil is a known carcinogen • Information regarding the health effects of refined mineral oils is still inconclusive • Derived from petroleum (see petroleum)
Nylon/rayon fibers	• Used in mascara as a thickener • Potential irritants, especially for contact lens wearers • Nonbiodegradable environmental pollutants
Phenylenediamine	• Permanent hair dye ingredient • Derived from coal tar (see coal tar) • Common irritant • May cause severe dermatitis and eye irritation
Parabens	• Common allergen • Mimics estrogen at high levels
PEG, ceteareth, polyethylene	• Often contaminated by 1,4 dioxane (see 1,4 dioxane)
Petro-chemicals	• A category of chemicals derived from petroleum in which the extraction and refining stages exacerbates pollution and climate change • Includes chemicals such as mineral oil, petroleum jelly, propylene glycol, and paraffin
Petroleum distillates	• Often contaminated with carcinogens • May cause allergies
Polyethylene microbeads	• Plastic • Nonbiodegradable environmental pollutants that persist in waterways and get ingested by wildlife
Silicones	• Nonbiodegradable environmental pollutants • Found persisting in waterways • Acts as a nonbreathable film over skin
Sodium lauryl sulfate	• Can cause severe epidermis changes • Irritant at 2% and greater • Common detergent in shampoos • May cause hair loss • May clog pores and hair follicles

Table 15-1. Beware of These Ingredients Cont'd

Ingredient	What's the catch?
Synthetic colors (D&C, FD&C)	• Chemical mixtures containing ingredients that may be carcinogenic; widespread use in many food types.
Toluene	• Chronic and acute toxicity in animals and humans • Causes central nervous system dysfunction and narcosis, leading to fatigue, headaches, nausea, etc.
Triclosan	• Hormone disrupters in animals • Further studies need to be done to understand effects on humans • Often found in antibacterial products (which are found to be no more effective than normal soap)
Urea	• May release formaldehyde (see formaldehyde)

For your ease of use, here is a similar guide that categorizes the above chemicals into the products they are typically found in (see Table 15-2):

Table 15-2. Cosmetics Shopping Guide

Product	Try to avoid using products containing...
For cleansing	
Face wash, body wash, shampoo	Sodium lauryl sulfate, fragrance, diethanolamine, triethanolamine
Exfoliators	Polyethylene or polypropylene (PP, PE, plastic) microbeads, fragrance
Hand soap	Triclosan often found in antibacterial soap, sodium lauryl sulfate, fragrance
Toothpaste	Triclosan
Shaving cream	DMDM hydantoin, fragrance, PEG/ceteareth/polyethylene, triclosan
For moisturizing	
Body/face lotion	Hydroquinone (usually in skin-lightening products), fragrance, petrochemicals such as mineral oil, petroleum jelly, propylene glycol, and paraffin, and silicones such as dimethicone and siloxanes
Lip balm	Petrochemicals such as mineral oil, petroleum jelly, propylene glycol, paraffin, and fragrance
For Tanning	
Sunscreen	Aerosol spray or powder sunscreen, fragrance

Table 15-2. Cosmetics Shopping Guide Cont'd

Product	Try to avoid products containing...
For makeup	
Lipstick	Lead
Nail polish	Formaldehyde, toluene, dibutyl phthalate (DBP)
Polish remover	Formaldehyde
Foundation	Loose powders, silicones such as dimethicone and siloxanes
Mascara	Eyelash tint containing silver compounds, petroleum distillates
Miscellaneous	
Chemical hair treatments	Avoid Keratin treatments and ingredients such as formaldehyde and lead
Perfume/cologne	Fragrance
Deodorant	Formaldehyde, fragrance
Permanent hair dyes	Minimize permanent hair dyes in general, but especially dark permanent hair dyes with para-phenylenediamine

If you have frequent adverse reactions to cosmetic products, try to avoid the following chemicals that were tested to be the most common allergens by the North American Contact Dermatitis Group:[24]

- nickel sulfate

- myroxilon pereirae (balsam of Peru)

- fragrance mix 1

- quaternium-15

- neomycin

- bacitracin

- formaldehyde

- cobalt chloride

- methyldibromoglutaronitrile/phenoxyethanol

- P-phenylenediamine

- potassium dichromate

- carba mix

- thiuram mix

- diazolidinylurea

- 2-brono-2-nitropropane-1,3-diol

If these lists are giving you a headache, keep calm and carry on. In the next few sections, you will learn how to take simpler steps toward finding safe and healthy products.

Less is More

Whenever I walk down the cosmetics isles at supermarkets or drugstores, I cannot help but be overwhelmed: foot balm, cuticle cream, skin salve, healing balm…. Do we really *need* all of this? To sell their products, companies often try to make you think that you need something when you might not. Therefore, you can often find effective products that work for multiple purposes at the same time.

For example, Dr. Bronner's does an incredible job at creating simple and multipurpose products as a brand. They even teach you how to put their Pure-Castile Liquid Soap to 18 different uses: facial soap, body soap, shampoo, shaving cream, and even household uses, such as dishwashing soap, detergent, all-purpose cleaner, fruits and veggies wash, and so on. Or, Josie Maran's Infinity Cream can be used on any part of your body or face to nourish chapped skin.

While simplifying your needs is a personal lifestyle choice, it can help you:

- declutter your home, which can make you less stressed;

- reduce the amount of packaging waste that you generate; and

- reduce your risks of having adverse skin reactions.

Table 15-3 on the next page lists some common products you may have always thought you needed along with some alternate options to help you simplify your self-care regimen.

Table 15-3. How to Simplify Your Self-Care Products

Simplify	How to simplify...
Foot balm, lip balm, hand and cuticle creams, dry skin creams, healing balm	All of these balms are used to treat extremely dry or chapped skin. Look for all-purpose body balms or invest in a bottle of versatile high-quality moisturizing oil (e.g., coconut oil or argan oil) to cover your needs.
Body soap, hand wash, antibacterial wash, wash for dry skin, etc.	The primary purpose of using soap is to cut grease and wash away impurities. While many of us pick antibacterial hand wash to prevent infectious diseases, common antibacterial soaps containing triclosan have been shown to be no more effective at keeping people healthy and at reducing bacterial levels than plain soap.[25] So, just stick to one type of soap or even just a bar soap, which reduces the need for plastic packaging. Add some all-purpose oil, such as argan oil or coconut oil, into the soap to treat dryer skin.
Body or face exfoliators	The purpose of using exfoliators is to get rid of dead skin cells. Unfortunately, conventional versions are often made with plastic microbeads, many of which end up bypassing wastewater treatments and contaminating our rivers and waterways. Use a luffa sponge or washcloth instead, or add some brown sugar or sea salt into your body wash and scrub away!
Shaving cream	The objective of using shaving cream is to soften your skin for a smoother shave. Simply add all-purpose oils, such as coconut oil, argan oil, shea butter, or other moisturizing oils into your regular soap and shave away!
Hair mask	Hair masks are used to give your hair an extra boost of hydration. Add some coconut oil or even a mashed avocado or other moisturizing oils into your regular conditioner and leave it in your hair for longer than usual before rinsing.
Face moisturizer, face gels, face creams, serums, face oils, whatever new names they give it...	The purpose of skin care products in general is to help maintain your skin's natural health and keep its own functions intact. Unless you have a special routine prescribed for your personal needs, keep your facial care products to a minimum, just enough to keep your skin hydrated, nourished, and protected.
Makeup and eye makeup remover	Makeup remover is often used to remove oil-based makeup that cannot be washed off by water. Try using high-quality, all-purpose oils, such as extra virgin olive oil or sunflower seed oil. These oils will effectively remove any oil-based makeup without your needing to worry about what chemicals may be in your makeup removers.

To make shopping for healthy cosmetic products less troublesome, you can also apply the "less is more" concept when skimming through a product's ingredient list. The simpler the list, the less the risk you run for any adverse reactions.

By choosing products with simpler ingredients, you also minimize what is called the "cocktail effect." (Unfortunately, the results are not as pleasant as at happy hours.) The "cocktail effect" in chemistry is the idea that chemicals can interact with one another to produce effects different from what they would have produced by themselves. Since chemicals are often only studied independently, the potentially undesirable effects of multiple chemicals working together are not well understood.[26]

For the most part, you will be perfectly fine using products with long and complicated ingredient lists. However, if you have sensitive skin and want to reduce your risks for any adverse reactions, pick products with simpler ingredients; they can be just as effective. No matter what products you end up choosing, however, keep in mind that even the simplest and purest of ingredients can give you allergic reactions. So, always test out new products daily for a week on the inner part of your elbow before applying them all over your body or face (see Chapter 17).

Chapter Summary

Questionable Until Proven Safe

What goes around comes around. Because our current wastewater treatment systems are not able to filter out all of the chemicals we pollute our waters with, dumping more untested or harmful chemicals into our waterways will just increase our own health risks. Let's focus on **problem prevention** and reduce the amount of products we buy that contain nonbiodegradable or shown/suspected harmful ingredients. This way, we can better target the problem at its roots.

Better Safe Than Sorry

Because marketing labels on cosmetic products such as "all natural" or "dermatologist tested" are unregulated, your best way of understanding what exactly is in a product is to read the list of ingredients. Whenever possible, try to avoid ingredients established or suspected to be harmful to humans, animals, or ecological health.

Less Is More

The less complicated the ingredient list and the fewer products you use, the safer you will be from any adverse reactions or chemical sensitivities. Plus, simplifying your self-care products can also help you save money, declutter your home, and decrease the amount of packaging waste you generate!

Chapter 16

Use Power for Good

One of the most impactful shopping decisions you can make is to support brands that value the three *Ps*: *People, Planet,* and *Profit*. These are three widely validated considerations that many responsible companies incorporate into their business practices.[27]

If you need a new bottle of lotion and have a choice between buying from a conventional company versus another that makes conscious efforts to minimize its impacts on the environment and to contribute to social welfare, choosing the latter benefits not only you and that company, but also the world, simply as an effortless, positive byproduct of your decision. Remember: You are the consumer, and you have power to drive little changes with every choice you make in life—yes, even through a mundane decision like picking which company to buy your shampoo from.

Responsible Brands Value People

Do companies really care about your health? Are they transparent about what ingredients they have used and what tests they have done? Do they care about their workers' safety? Even if certain ingredients are safe at levels found in the final product but are suspected or established carcinogens at higher doses, responsible companies would still try to avoid using these ingredients to ensure the safety of people that regularly come in contact with large quantities of these chemicals (e.g., cosmetologists, people who work in cosmetics factories).

Does the company take part in any charitable events or support social or environmental causes? If production is outsourced to a foreign country, does the company show signs of caring about its supply chain and workers abroad? These are just some questions you can try to answer to see if a brand values the health of its customers and workers.

Responsible Brands Value Our Planet

Responsible brands think about their impacts in everything they do. They value:

- sourcing sustainable ingredients;

- minimizing impacts during production;

- minimizing toxic byproducts and wastes;

- using more eco-friendly packaging materials; and

- communicating all of this with their consumers, who have a right to know their products' history.

For example, The Honest Company excels at communicating how it is making its products safer and healthier for its consumers. Not only does it openly reveal what ingredients are used, what for, and where they come from, but it also takes care to package its goods with environmentally conscious materials.

Often, companies that value our planet are also the same ones that end up using more natural or organic ingredients, because they value the powers of nature and have chosen to advocate a lifestyle more closely connected to our natural environment. For example, Earth Tu Face creates skincare products made with 100% plant-based, food grade ingredients based on its belief that "[you should never put] on your skin what you would not put in your mouth."[28] While some may call this extreme, skin-care products made with food-grade ingredients may be as healthy and as eco-friendly as they can get.

If you are making a personal choice to use more natural or organic cosmetic products, just beware of green-washing. Companies that use eco-friendly marketing statements simply to sell more products, while not actually living up to their claimed standards or missions, are said to be *green-washing*. As always, skip any unregulated marketing statements (e.g., "all natural," "eco-friendly," "sustainable"), and try to obtain more objective information, for example, by reading the list of ingredients, or by looking for certifications from third-party organizations. While there are numerous types of organic certifications (see Table 16-1, below), each with their own quality standards, these indicators generally have more credibility than any unsupported claims that were made from the company alone.

Table 16-1. Well-known Organizations That Certify Organic Cosmetics

Organization Name	Certification
US Department of Agriculture	USDA Organic
American National Standards Institute	NSF/ANSI 305
Organic and Sustainable Industry Standards	OASIS Organic
Ecocert of France	Ecocert
Australian Certified Organic Standard	Australian Organic
Soil Association Certification (U.K.)	Soil Association Organic

In determining whether a brand is concerned about the environment, you can also look at what materials it uses to package its products; the less of it used, the better. Some of the most eco-friendly packaging options are ones made from recycled or biodegradable materials, such as recycled glass, recycled plastic, or post-consumer recycled cardboard packaging.

Amber Hawthorne, founder of Bambu Earth, has taken this another step further by creating bar-soap packaging that is not only biodegradable but will even grow into a flower when planted in the soil—from trash into a blooming flower! Imagine if every packaging we had in the world took after this model…our landfills would become botanical gardens!

Responsible Brands Need Our Support

For any business to be sustainable, it must be profitable. For charitable businesses to continue to make their positive contributions to the world, they must profit, too. To do so, they openly communicate their good practices with conscious consumers like you who support those businesses that are using their power to drive positive change in our world.

Get to know whether the brand behind your products values the three *Ps* by looking through their social media pages, websites, product descriptions, certifications, and so on. If you are too busy to look through long lists of ingredients and to research stories behind every brand, however, you can begin by shopping at retailers that value our health and the health of our planet (e.g., The Organic Project, Credo Beauty, LeVert Beauty, Mindful Luxe, etc.). Since these retailers uphold similar values to ours, they will most likely (and hopefully) have done the proper research when choosing which products to stock for their customers.

Chapter Summary

Responsible Brands Value People

Responsible brands value people's health—within their local communities, of their consumers, their employees, and workers and cosmetologists who come into contact with large doses of their products. Therefore, they minimize their use of known or suspected toxic chemicals whenever possible.

Responsible Brands Value Our Planet

Responsible brands care about the health of our planet. So they do everything in their power to minimize their environmental impact. They aim to source sustainable, biodegradable, and nontoxic ingredients; package their products using eco-conscious materials; and source local ingredients and materials whenever possible.

Responsible Brands Need Our Support

Responsible brands need to profit in order to continue to use their power for good. Therefore, they try to communicate their good practices to you. When looking for an eco- and people-friendly product, ask questions and try to look for objective information regarding their products and business practices (i.e., list of ingredients, certifications, packaging material, causes they support, etc.).

Chapter 17

Mind Your Skin

Your skin contains billions of living cells that work continuously to maintain your dermal health. It serves many important functions, such as naturally detoxing itself, secreting oils to seal in hydration, regulating body temperature, reacting to allergens or harsh chemicals as a warning to avoid certain substances, and so on. However, because your mind, body, and surrounding environment can all affect your skin's natural functions, living a holistically healthy lifestyle is a crucial first step toward beautifying your skin from the inside out.

To recap what has been discussed thus far: living healthy holistically includes taking care of your mental well-being; getting regular physical activity and quality sleep; eating a balanced diet and staying hydrated; and, overall, making more eco-conscious choices to reduce the amount of environmental stressors (air pollution, water pollution, toxic wastes, etc.) to which you personally contribute and expose yourself.

On top of all of this, however, you can benefit from becoming more attentive to your skin's condition and adopting a self-care routine that helps enhance and protect its natural functions.

Squeaky Clean Can Damage Your Skin

People often feel that washing until they are "squeaky-clean" is the proper way to keep their skin clear and healthy. However, the natural oils produced by our skin are not "dirty," and scrubbing our skin will not make acne or skin irritations go away. In fact, the safest and most natural skin moisturizers are the oils produced by our own bodies. They are naturally secreted to seal in hydration and protect our skin from environmental stressors.

Therefore, scrubbing and deep-cleansing too often (even for oily skin) can disrupt its natural barriers, causing it to become more sensitive or irritated over time. While you should definitely remove excess oil, sweat, dirt, and other impurities from your skin, do so *gently* so you will not harm your skin cells during the process.

When asked how to properly wash the skin during showers without irritating it, dermatologist Sandra T. Yeh, MD FAAD suggested:

- Limit showers to 3-5 minutes long.

- Do not use hot water for showers.

- After showering, pat dry (instead of rubbing dry) with a towel.

- After drying, apply cream to seal in hydration.

To best maintain your facial hygiene without damaging your skin, try to regularly use gentle cleansers, deep cleanse only once in a while, and change your pillowcases often.

Don't Let the Sunshine Make You Whine

Skin cancer caused by UV rays has increased year after year in the past decade, and an estimated one in five Americans will develop skin cancer in his or her lifetime.[29] In addition, one's risk for melanoma, the deadliest type of skin cancer, increases by a shocking 50% with just five or more sunburn incidences.[30]

To keep your skin well protected, avoid being in the sun between its peak hours of 10:00 a.m. to 2:00 p.m., use sunscreen, wear hats and cover-ups, and seek shade when your skin begins to turn red. Getting burnt and having your skin peel neither looks nor feels sexy, despite how hot you will feel, literally.

A Lively Organ

Like for our diets, there are no perfect skin care regimens that work for everybody. Everyone's bodies are different, and everyone's skin types are different, too. So get to know your own skin and its needs, and then use trial and error to find products most suitable for you.

If you are introducing a new product into your self-care routine, patch-test it first on the skin inside of your elbows once a day for a week—even if it is labeled "all natural," "dermatologist tested," "hypoallergenic," etc. If you experience any adverse reactions, immediately and completely abandon the new product. Otherwise, you should be able to start using it safely on other parts of your body without concern. Keep in mind, however, that some reactions happen after chronic long-term use, and new skin allergies can develop as you age. Therefore, continue to watch for signs of irritation after using a new product for a few weeks, or even several months.

To best protect your skin's natural functions, try to be more mindful of your skin's signals to you, and make sure you react accordingly. For example, if your skin is becoming irritated for any reason, take a break from your usual skin-care routine and use only mild cleansers and simple hydrating creams for a few days. Or, if your skin is starting to turn bright red from too much sun exposure, seek shade, and drink lots of water.

Remember: Your skin is not a dead surface. It is full of life, constantly working to balance, detox, and maintain itself. Your role to help protect and enhance its natural functions is simply to become attentive to its signals to you; to take care of your mind, body, and surrounding environment holistically; and to adopt a simple, healthy skin-care routine that will best address its needs.

Chapter Summary

Squeaky Clean Can Damage Your Skin

To keep the natural functions of your skin intact, do not overwash and overexfoliate your skin. Keep your showers under five minutes, do not wash with hot water, pat (instead of rub) your skin dry, and put on creams immediately after drying to seal in hydration. To maintain good facial hygiene, change your pillowcases often, wash regularly with mild cleansers, and don't use deep cleansers too often.

Don't Let the Sunshine Make You Whine

To have fun safely in the sun, avoid being outside for extended amounts of time during the sun's peak hours between 10 a.m.–2 p.m. Additionally, use sun protection, wear cover-ups and hats, stay hydrated, and seek shade, especially when your skin begins to turn red.

A Lively Organ

Skin is your body's largest organ, and it is full of living cells constantly working to balance, detox, and maintain themselves. So, to keep your skin healthy holistically, you will need to become attentive to its needs, adopt a simple and healthy skin-care regimen suitable for your specific skin type, and take care of your mind, body, and environment holistically.

Part References

1   Thibodeau, G. A., & Patton, K. T. (2011). *Structure & function of the body* (14th ed.). St. Louis, MO: Elsevier Mosby.

2   Natural Resources Defense Council. (n.d.). *Protecting people from unsafe chemicals*. Retrieved from http://www.nrdc.org/health/toxics.asp

3   President's Cancer Panel. (2010). *Reducing environmental cancer risk* (Rep.). Bethesda, MD: US Department of Health and Human Services. Retrieved from http://deainfo.nci.nih.gov/advisory/pcp/annualReports/pcp08-09rpt/PCP_Report_08-09_508.pdf

4   Environmental Working Group. (n.d.). Exposures add up – Survey results. Retrieved from http://www.ewg.org/skindeep/2004/06/15/exposures-add-up-survey-results/

5   Centers for Disease Control and Prevention. (2012, April 30). *Skin exposures and effects*. Retrieved from http://www.cdc.gov/niosh/topics/skin/

6   Liu, X., Ji, K., & Choi, K. (2012). Endocrine disruption potentials of organo-phosphate flame retardants and related mechanisms in H295R and MVLN cell lines and in zebrafish. *Aquatic Toxicology, 114-115*, 173-181.

7   Mendelsohn, E., Hagopian, A., Hoffman, K., Butt, C. M., Lorenzo, A., Congleton, J., . . . Stapleton, H. M. (2016). Nail polish as a source of exposure to triphenyl phosphate. *Environment International, 86*, 45-51.

8   Concin, N., Hofstetter, G., Plattner, B., Tomovski, C., Fiselier, K., Gerritzen, K., . . . Grob, K. (2011). Evidence for cosmetics as a source of mineral oil contamination in women. *Journal of Women's Health, 20*(11), 1713-1719.

9   Groot, A. C., & White, I. R. (2001). Cosmetics and skin care products. Ed. Richard J. G. Rycroft. In *Textbook of contact dermatitis*, 661-685.

10 Dolan, L. C., Matulka, R. A., & Burdock, G. A. (2010). Naturally occurring food toxins. *Toxins, 2*(9), 2289-2332.

11 Trautmann, N. (2005). *The dose makes the poison—or does it?* American Institute of Biological Sciences. Retrieved from http://www.actionbioscience.org/

12 Natural Resources Defense Council. (n.d.). *Protecting people from unsafe chemicals*. Retrieved from http://www.nrdc.org/health/toxics.asp

13 Donald, J. M., Hooper, K., & Hopenhayn-Rich, C. (1991). Reproductive and developmental toxicity of toluene: A review. *Environmental Health Perspectives, 94*, 237.

14 Donald, J. M., Hooper, K., & Hopenhayn-Rich, C. (1991). Reproductive and developmental toxicity of toluene: A review. *Environmental Health Perspectives, 94,* 237.

15 Natural Resources Defense Council. (2013). *An introduction to federal environmental policy.* Retrieved from http://www.nrdc.org/legislation/policy-basics/files/policy-basics-full.pdf

16 Luntz, T. (2009, December 14). *US drinking water widely contaminated.* Retrieved from http://www.scientificamerican.com/article/tap-drinking-water-contaminants-pollutants/

17 International Joint Commission. (2000). *Protection of the waters of the Great Lakes: Final report to the governments of Canada and the United States* (Rep.). Retrieved from http://www.ijc.org/files/publications/ID1560.pdf

18 Drinan, J., Spellman, F. R., & Drinan, J. (2013). *Water and wastewater treatment: A guide for the nonengineering professional.* Boca Raton, FL: CRC Press.

19 Concin, N., Hofstetter, G., Plattner, B., Tomovski, C., Fiselier, K., Gerritzen, K., . . . Grob, K. (2011). Evidence for cosmetics as a source of mineral oil contamination in women. *Journal of Women's Health, 20*(11), 1713-1719.

20 Personal Care Products Council. (n.d.). *Cosmetics info: The science & safety behind your favorite products.* Retrieved November, 2015, from http://www.cosmeticsinfo.org/

21 Environmental Working Group. (n.d.). *EWG's skin deep® cosmetics database.* Retrieved November, 2015, from http://www.ewg.org/skindeep/

22 U.S. Environmental Protection Agency. (n.d.) *Safer Chemicals Research.* Retrieved November, 2015, from http://www.epa.gov/chemical-research

23 U.S. Food and Drug Administration. (n.d.) Chemical contaminants. Retrieved November, 2015, from http://www.fda.gov/food/foodborneillnesscontaminants/chemicalcontaminants/default.htm

24 Zug, K. A., Warshaw, E. M., Fowler, J. F., Jr., Maibach, H. I., Belsito, D. L., Pratt, M. D., . . . Marks, J. (2009). Patch-test results of the North American Contact Dermatitis Group 2005-2006. *Dermatitis, 30*(3), 149-160.

25 Aiello, A. E., Larson, E. L., & Levy, S. B. (2007). Consumer antibacterial soaps: Effective or just risky? *Clinical Infectious Diseases, 45*(S2), S137-S147.

26 European Commission. (2015). *Combination effects of chemicals,* Environment—European Commission. Retrieved from http://ec.europa.eu/environment/chemicals/effects/effects_en.htm

27   Rinaldi, F. R., & Testa, S. (2014). *The responsible fashion company: Integrating ethics and aesthetics in the supply chain.* Sheffield: Greenleaf Publishing, p22

28   Earth Tu Face (n.d.) About Earth Tu Face. Retrieved from http://www.earthtuface.com/pages/about-us

29   Robinson, J. K. (2005). Sun exposure, sun protection, and vitamin D. *Jama, 294*(12), 1541.

30   Pfahlberg, A., Kölmel, K. F., & Gefeller, O. (2001). Timing of excessive ultraviolet radiation and melanoma: Epidemiology does not support the existence of a critical period of high susceptibility to solar ultraviolet radiation-induced melanoma. *British Journal of Dermatology, 144*(3), 471-475.

PART V

STYLE

"Every drop in the ocean counts."

—Yoko Ono

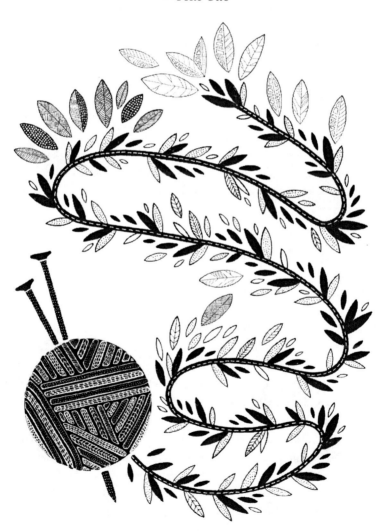

Chapter 18

Dress Without Stripping Our Planet

There is no denying that we are visual creatures. We are simply drawn to things that are attractive: flattering tops, sleek dress shirts, eye-catching accessories, and so on. On the surface, your shopping choices may appear to be very innocent: you go to a store, pick out a shirt you fancy, and check out at the register before being able to proudly claim it as yours. However, that five-minute decision means much, much more than you think, because your shirt is not just a shirt.

It also embodies the story of its entire journey: where the raw materials came from, what the working conditions were like for the farmers and workers involved, how much toxic chemicals were used for manufacturing, how far it traveled throughout this entire process, and so on. Unfortunately, without your even realizing it, the innocent act of buying a shirt can result in your support for labor abuse, unfair trade, social injustice, occupational health hazards for farmers and factory workers, detrimental environmental impacts, contamination of your drinking water, and so on. Alas, the fashion industry is not as glamorous as it appears.

An Ugly Industry Masked by Pretty Things

The textiles industry is one of the largest polluters on earth, and it is also the fifth-largest contributor to carbon dioxide emissions in the United States.[1,2] Unfortunately, these levels are even higher in other regions of the world where economies are reliant on textiles manufacturing. In addition, the industry as a whole is extremely wasteful; energy, water, and chemically intensive; and because of the often long, complex supply chain from production to the final product, not as well regulated as it could and should be.

You might ask: How is it possible that we as consumers can be working against the very social and environmental issues we care about? The answer is similar to what has happened to our food culture: we have become disconnected from the stories behind all of this "stuff." Many of us have no idea what polyester is made of, how cotton is grown, what chemicals are used to fabricate our clothing, who makes our clothes, and how far these products have traveled from their origins to their final destinations. And we are not alone; 91% of companies do not even know where all of their cotton fiber comes from, and 75% do not know the source of all of their fabrics and materials.[3]

This disconnect between us and the histories behind our daily consumer products has led us to make decisions we did not know were self-destructive. But it doesn't have to be this way. It's time for us to reconnect with the origins of our stuff, and it's time for us to reconnect with our natural environment through our consumer choices. After all, anything that concerns our health and the health of our planet deserves our attention and care.

The "Slow Fashion" Movement

Traditionally, the fashion cycle took around 18 months from design, material sourcing, CTM (cutting, trimming, and making), to retail. Many designer or slow fashion brands follow a similar timeline today. However, the invention of "fast fashion" by brands such as Zara and H&M has completely transformed the fashion cycle. Rather than offering the traditional seasonal collections, fast-fashion brands bring new styles of clothing into their stores every single week! Instead of inspiring people to appreciate design and craftsmanship and encouraging people to cherish their clothes more, fast fashion often just seduces its consumers into becoming more and more consumptive.

To keep prices as low as possible, many fashion brands have also exported manufacturing to developing countries where many laborers are underpaid, working conditions are not up to acceptable safety standards, children are illegally employed, and highly toxic chemicals banned in industrialized countries are still in use.

On April 24, 2013, a tragic accident occurred in Bangladesh. An eight-story commercial building containing several garment factories that manufactured clothes for big brands such as Benetton, Primark, and Wal-Mart collapsed from structural failure. This tragic accident led to more than a thousand deaths and thousands more injured. When cracks were discovered in the building the day beforehand, the shops and banks in the building immediately closed down. However, the garment workers were ordered to return to work despite the safety hazard.

Unfortunately, the lack of stringent regulations in developing countries, the lack of transparency in the industry, as well as the disconnect between key players in the supply chain all make it extremely difficult to improve the working conditions for the many workers who are silently abused behind the scenes. The cheap price tags of many fashion products are simply *not* reflective of their real costs: environmental costs from air and water pollution and the improper treatment of chemical waste; social costs from unsafe working conditions, labor abuse and child labor; and global health costs from damages to our planet's health.

Of course, not all fast-fashion products or products with cheap price tags are made in unhealthy ways. For example, even though H&M is a fast-fashion brand, it has taken notable and important steps in the past few years toward making its supply chain more transparent and its products more sustainable (e.g., using more eco-friendly materials and supporting nonprofit organizations). However, the numerous problems associated with the fashion industry as a whole still underscore the importance of us looking past a product's physical properties and price tag when we shop.

Instead of quantity, we must focus on *quality.* Instead of merely judging a product by its appearance, we must shed light on its history. Instead of getting caught up with the consumptive mindset fast fashion encourages, we need to cherish every piece of clothing we own and support "slow fashion," a movement emphasizing fair trade, fair wages, high-quality materials, handmade artisan work, and the intelligent blend of traditional knowledge with modern technology.

Your Decisions Matter

We are disgusted by polluted rivers and lakes. We frown in disapproval upon articles discussing social injustice. We shake our heads at the increasingly alarming statistics on climate change. But, above all, we feel completely helpless, as we are so far removed from all of these global problems.

But are we really *that* far removed? If we trace back many of the above issues, it becomes clear that we, whether we realize it or not, contribute to them through many of our seemingly innocent decisions.

Even if we all are not directly harmed by the toxic chemicals that are used, or the freshwater sources that are drained on the other side of the world, the resulting environmental impact will come around and affect us sooner or later. As discussed in Chapter 4, everything is interconnected in our modern world, and Mother Nature knows no boundaries. The depletion of our planet's resources, no matter where, can increase global stress and conflict. Moreover, because housing costs near factories (along with their hazardous emissions and wastes) are much lower than elsewhere, many struggling below the poverty line often have no choice but to live in these hazardous zones. Therefore, threatening the clean water, fresh air, and food security of any given region in the world not only contributes to *regional* environmental issues; it also aggravates *global* environmental, social justice, and human and animal rights issues as well.

Suddenly, there are so many new things to think about. Could your previous purchases have contributed to some social or environmental problem you read about in the newspaper? Does this make you evil? Well, of course not! No one goes shopping with the intention of hurting anyone. Helene Serignac, a French TV journalist who focuses on eco-fashion, noted it is natural that we ask ourselves only these three questions when we go shopping for clothes:

1. Will I look good in this?

2. Is it comfortable?

3. Can I afford it?

However, now that you are aware of the potential problems your purchases may be supporting, I urge you to add another question to that list: "What is this product's *impact*?" Think about what social and environmental impacts the product could have had before landing in your hands, what impacts it may create during your ownership, and what impacts it will go on to have after you throw it away. There are so many questions to think about, and you may not be able to answer all of them right away. But by beginning to ask these important questions, you can influence the way companies plan and make their new products. After all, companies thrive by satisfying the desires and needs of their consumers.

When you begin to see that you (as a consumer) play a key role in shaping a company's future direction, you might just realize how much your voice and your choices matter. And once you are aware of the dark side of the fashion industry, there is no turning back; shopping might never feel the same again.

Instead of focusing on all of the scary problems you may contribute to, however, let's look at the bright side. Take a moment and think about all of the positive impacts you can bolster, just by making more informed decisions. You, my reader, have the power to help make our world a better place through your fashion choices in ways including helping to:

• Fight for social and environmental justice;

• Fight against labor abuse and child labor;

• Reduce water and air pollution;

- Decrease occupational health hazards for farmers and workers;

- Decrease your health risks from toxic chemical residues on clothing;

- Reduce the amount of accumulating, nonbiodegradable trash on our planet.

Isn't it eye-opening that something so mundane can be so meaningful? And isn't it exciting to know that you can look good, do good, and feel good at the same time? With all of this in mind, it is time to translate these motivations into action. What does *mindful shopping* mean when it comes down to decision-making? In the next few chapters, you will learn how to become a responsible shopper of fashion and home products. As a start, however, just keep in mind that a shirt is more than a shirt, and a tie is more than a tie. Everything you see within stores has a history waiting to be unraveled.

Chapter Summary

An Ugly Industry Masked by Pretty Things

Unfortunately, the fashion industry behind the scene is not all that glamorous. There are many social and environmental problems associated with the fashion industry, including child labor; underpaid labor; air and water pollution; intensive water, chemical, and energy use; unsafe working conditions; and health risks for consumers. Therefore, we need to begin to unveil the histories of our daily consumer products, rather than simply judging them based on their appearances.

The "Slow Fashion" Movement

Rather than getting caught up with the consumptive mindset encouraged by **fast fashion** (which often uses cheap labor, cheap materials, and irresponsible practices to maximize profits), we need to cherish our clothes and shift our focus to **slow fashion**, which values handmade artisan work, high-quality raw materials, fair wages, and fair trade.

Your Decisions Matter

Despite how complex and powerful the fashion industry is, the companies are powerless without their consumers' support. Through voicing our concerns and making more conscious purchasing decisions, we have the collective power to drive positive change in the industry.

Chapter 19

Trash-Talk

Meet the Pacific Trash Vortex, a massive patch of floating garbage, pollutants, plastics, chemical sludge, and other debris circling in the currents of the Pacific Ocean. Although it is difficult to determine the exact size of this patch because many of the contaminants cannot be seen by the human eye, it is estimated to range from the size of Texas to many more times that size. But this is not even the only garbage patch out there in our oceans. According to the 5 Gyres Organization, similar ones have accumulated in all of the other major oceans as well.

What is so disheartening is the finding from 1997 that 44% of all species of sea birds, 86% of all species of sea turtles, and 43% of all species of marine mammals were known to ingest plastic.[4,5] If plastic debris accumulates and blocks the digestive tracts of our marine creatures, they can suffocate and starve to death. Oh, and a quarter of the fish tested in markets within the United States were found to contain ingested man-made debris, some of which were plastic.[6] To make matters worse, because of the massive quantities of pollutants we regularly dump into our natural environments, our fish are also very likely to be contaminated with a cocktail of potentially harmful chemicals.[7,8] "Shrimp chemical cocktail" for lunch, anyone?

How did all of this happen? Alarmingly, we generate massive amounts of trash from every aspect of our lives—fashion being a major one of them. Livia Firth, founder of Eco Age and executive producer of *The True Cost*, noted that, on average, fast fashion pieces last for only *five weeks* within a consumer's wardrobe before being tossed out. The Environmental Protection Agency (EPA) also reports that the average American throws away more than 68 pounds of clothing and textiles every year![9] Unfortunately, when we buy into this faster and faster, cheaper and cheaper mentality of fast fashion, we are also aggravating many of our world's problems faster and faster. Instead of being lured into this vicious cycle, it helps to take a step back to examine what is really happening on a larger scale.

Keep in Mind What's out of Sight

Where exactly does our trash go after garbage trucks come to pick it up? Some is recycled, some incinerated, some composted. However, most of it ends up being piled into our landfills of trash-mountains. And then what happens? It sits there for years, decades, and centuries, reeking and leaking contaminants into our lands, water, and air. Our current waste system is simply out of balance. The rate at which we add to our trash piles is much faster than the rate at which they are able to break down naturally or are artificially treated in some way.

By examining the way natural ecosystems function, it becomes clear that the creation of waste in and of itself is completely normal. However, within every sustainable system, one's waste always goes on to become something of value to another in an ongoing cycle. For example, an animal's wastes, such as food scraps and feces, get broken down into soil nutrients by microorganisms. These nutrients are then taken up by plants to facilitate their growth, thus continually recycling the animal's wastes back into the circle of life.

As another example, plants produce oxygen as their waste, but oxygen is what animals need to survive. On the flipside, animals breathe out carbon dioxide as "waste," but this waste is what plants need to grow. So, you might ask, why has carbon dioxide been demonized if this waste is actually considered food for plants? The reason is because there is now an *imbalance* of it within our atmosphere, and the continually increasing concentration of carbon dioxide is directly and indirectly causing various harmful consequences to our planet (i.e., climate change, ocean acidification, increased prevalence of mosquito-borne diseases, etc.).

As you can see, the fact that we produce trash is not problematic. The problems are the rate at which we throw things out and the types of trash we generate.

Some garbage made with natural materials will readily break down in the environment within a few weeks, months, or years (leftover food, fabrics made from natural fibers, our biological waste, etc.). This type of trash is not as troublesome as it works with the ways our natural world functions. Whether it contains toxic chemical residues that may seep into our lands, however, is another story.

While products made with synthetic materials might not be able to naturally break down for centuries, some can be recycled indefinitely. Glass expert and engineer Wei-Ching Liao notes that glass can be reprocessed again and again into new glass products without losing its original chemical structure, thus making it a relatively sustainable material. However, the same cannot be said for plastic. Because plastic degenerates when recycled, it will eventually degrade to the point where it can no longer be recycled again. Therefore, with our current recycling technology, most plastic products will still add to our persisting piles of trash when they are disposed of—even if they are labeled "recyclable."

Perhaps even more cumbersome are the many products made with *mixtures* of biodegradable and non-biodegradable components (e.g., a knitted shirt with 50% cotton and 50% polyester). If the two parts are difficult to separate, the product will not be able to go through the natural biodegradation route or the artificial recycling path. Michael Braungart and William McDonough, authors of *Cradle to Cradle,* named such products "monstrous hybrids" because of how troublesome they are to dispose of.[10]

So, how can we begin to address our appalling mountains of garbage and trash vortexes that are only growing larger by the second? On the one hand, we need to support organizations working to clean up the mess we have already created. On the other hand, we also need to address the problem at its roots. As mentioned previously, we need to *slow down* the pace at which we throw things out. Therefore, we need to cherish more the things we already own and emphasize quality over quantity in the new things we buy. Whenever possible, we also need to prioritize products made with either 100% biodegradable or indefinitely recyclable materials.

Reduce: Less is More

To reduce the shocking amount of trash each of us generates, we need to rethink our consumer decisions. While completely abandoning consumerism may not be a practical solution, it is still important for us to shift our focus from quantity to quality. Look for clothing that will last you 5, 10, 20 years—perhaps even durable and classic enough to be passed down in your family for generations. Or, as Firth suggests, buy only clothing you will end up wearing at least 30 times. Save the money you would have spent on 5 or 10 cheap fashion items, and invest it in one high-quality piece instead.

To help you reduce the amount you buy—therefore, the amount you eventually throw out—ask yourself the following questions before buying something:

- Do I need this? Can I live without this? Can I wait a few days to see how badly I want it?

- Where will this item be in 1 year? 5 years? 10?

- Is the material high quality, or will it tear in a few washes?

- Will the style go out of fashion in a season? Or is it a classic piece that can be worn year after year?

- What is this item made of? Will I potentially be contributing to social, environmental, and global health issues by buying it?

When you become more mindful of what you buy and start to think twice before taking something to the cashier, you might just realize how many times you end up putting something back. After all, saving up to buy a high-quality jacket made responsibly by a happy, healthy human being is likely to make the purchase feel more fulfilling than if you were to buy 10 pieces made from cheap labor and unhealthy materials.

Long-Lasting Materials, Long-Lasting Issues

If you look within typical fashion stores—especially fast-fashion chains—you will see that a large portion of their clothing is made of synthetic materials such as polyester, nylon, and acrylic. Why are these fibers so prevalent? Because they are made from cheap petroleum-based chemicals and are long-lasting. However, the combination of fashion being cheap and nonbiodegradable is a dangerous one. Because clothes made from these materials are cheap, the volume of these clothes made, bought, and then tossed out will skyrocket. And because of their inability to biodegrade, the amount of persisting trash we generate will also skyrocket.

Unfortunately, the manufacture of polyester and other synthetic fabrics also requires heavy energy input and releases emissions such as volatile organic compounds, particulate matter, and acid gases—all of which can lead to respiratory disease.[11] Therefore, the more we support cheap, unhealthy fashion, the faster and more seriously we will poison our planet and ourselves.

With better incentives and improving technology, perhaps manufacturers will be able to cut down on their environmental impacts. And with increased consumer awareness, perhaps people will learn to cherish their clothes more before responsibly disposing of them. Even so, another lesser-known global problem—*microplastic pollution*—can still be aggravated by the mere existence of these nonbiodegradable fabrics.

Every time we wash our clothes, they shed tiny fibers into the water, bypass wastewater treatments because of their minuscule size, and then enter our rivers, lakes, and oceans. When ecologist Mark Browne, PhD, and his research team tossed clothes into a washing machine, they found that a garment can shed more than 1,900 microfibers per wash.[12] Not to their surprise, 18 of the 18 beaches they tested around the world were contaminated by microplastics, the majority consisting of polyester and acrylic microfibers.[13]

While plastic fibers shed from clothing are not the only sources of microplastic pollution, Browne's study suggests they are major ones. Unlike lint shed from natural fabrics, microplastic fibers do not break down in nature and may end up being consumed by wild animals, ingested by the fish that may wind up on our dinner plates, or inhaled and ingested by people as dust. And, although the long-term effects of microplastic contamination within natural environments are still being studied, they are known to release chemicals toxic to wildlife (i.e., bisphenol A or BPA, phthalates, nonylphenol, etc.), which can then enter our human diet.[14-16] Due to how hard it would be to execute large-scale global cleanups of marine debris and soil contamination, scientists and environmentalists alike stress the importance of urgently addressing this problem from its source. That is, we need to take a more *preventative* approach to confronting plastic and microplastic pollution.

For the manufacture of many products, plastic can be a very versatile, fitting choice of material. As our recycling facilities advance, we will also be able to more efficiently and effectively recycle used plastic products. So, for solid objects made of plastic, we simply need to reduce, reuse, and recycle properly so they do not pollute our oceans and lands.

However, for products made with microplastic fibers—which will inevitably shed from their source fabrics—we need to cut down on the amount that is manufactured in the first place. So, as fashion consumers, we need to minimize the amount of clothing we buy made with new, nonbiodegradable synthetic fibers (polyester, acrylic, nylon, etc.). We also need to use as long and frequently as possible our already existing nonbiodegradable clothing (to keep them out of landfills) and to dispose of them properly afterward. Rather than first trashing our world and then deciding how to clean up the mess, cutting down on the amount of nonbiodegradable clothing we produce and buy today (and throw away tomorrow) is a more sustainable solution that targets the problem at its roots.

Thankfully, as research and development continue, the number of healthier alternatives to nonrenewable and nonbiodegradable textiles will only increase. For example, for many years, sportswear companies relied on using neoprene— an energy-intensive, petroleum-based textile—to make wetsuits. However, Patagonia recently partnered with Yulex to develop a plant-based wetsuit material to lessen the environmental impacts of producing neoprene.

Technology has also allowed the development of biopolymers such as polylactic acid (PLA), a type of thermoplastic polyester made from 100% renewable sources like corn. Although PLA is not perfect, and its environmental impacts are still being assessed, it is less problematic to dispose of than conventional plastic would be, because it is biodegradable.

Finally, recycled polyethylene terephtalate (rPET), also known as recycled polyester, is another eco-friendlier alternative to conventional polyester, because it is made from recycled plastic bottles. Even though rPET fabrics can still shed microplastic fibers, its production is less energy-intensive, it helps to divert plastic trash away from landfills, and it converts waste into something of value again.

Keep it Simple

When you read about the special properties of textiles on their labels—flame-retardant, stain-resistant, wrinkle-free, odor-resistant, permanent press, antistatic, etc.—beware. This usually means that synthetic chemicals, often ones that will cause adverse reactions, were used to finish the fabric. While tags on clothing are required to show the material composition of the fabrics, they do not tell you what dyes and chemicals were used to process the clothing, or whether any chemical residues are left from production. However, the chemical treatments used on clothing often require heavy water usage, are poisonous to the workers, can cause adverse reactions in the consumers, and can produce effluent waste toxic to wildlife.[17]

Shockingly, over half of the 27 tested luxury children's clothing from brands such as Dior, Dolce & Gabbana, and Hermès were found to contain one or more hazardous chemical residues.[18] These chemicals include nonylphenol ethoxylates (NPEs), which break down into chemicals that are both toxic and bioaccumulative (will build up within organisms); and polyfluorinated chemicals (PFCs), which do not break down in the environment, bioaccumulate in the food chain, act as hormone disruptors, and are potentially carcinogenic.[19] If these findings don't already raise some red flags, according to a 2010 investigation by Beijing's Bureau of Industry and Commerce, more than half of the tested clothing brands in China—many of which were exported to the United States and other Western countries—"were found to contain toxic dyes that are known cancer-causing agents, or they failed to meet other basic quality standards."[20]

Although more concrete research is needed for us to better understand the health effects of exposures to the various chemical residues from our clothing, we do know that "As synthetic clothing dyes and garment finishes became more common and widespread on store shelves, so did the variety of reported health problems and chemical sensitivities experienced by ever-greater numbers of people of all ages."[21] As discussed in Part 4, many of the chemicals used to manufacture and finish our consumer goods are untested, so we have really become guinea pigs in a gigantic, global experiment. The beautiful glow of new clothes, their vibrant, mesmerizing colors, their silky smooth textures—are they really just beautifully poisonous?

Since we currently have little to no way of knowing what dyes or chemicals are used to manufacture our clothing from their tags (i.e., unless the information is voluntarily provided or the product has relevant certifications, such as the Oeko-Tex® Standard 100), we need to begin asking these questions. Just as we need to unveil the processes of the production of our food, we need to do the same for our fashion goods as well. As for now, while manufacturers work toward adopting healthier practices on the back end (reducing water usage, recycling water, air-dyeing textiles, using natural finishes, etc.), we can apply the "less is more" principle to the properties of our clothing in order to be safe rather than sorry. The simpler the finish, the safer we will be from potential health threats, and the safer our planet will be, too.

They Persist a While and Might Make You Infertile

Although our understandings of the potential health effects of wearing clothing made with different textiles are still limited, research so far suggests that wearing synthetic clothing may have undesired effects to the wearers. A study on contact dermatitis found that the clothes most likely to trigger adverse reactions were the synthetic ones finished with dispersive dark blue, brown, or black dyes.[22] Meanwhile, cotton and silk clothing rarely caused reactions. Another study found that polyester clothing altered the muscle activity of its wearers in a way that potentially caused muscle fatigue.[23,24] Although the specific reason is still unclear, researchers hypothesize that the electrostatic potential of the fabric might interfere with normal bodily functions.

To take this discussion on a slight tangent, even dogs wearing loose polyester underwear over 24 months had significantly lower sperm counts as a result.[25] Meanwhile, both the group wearing loose cotton underwear and the control group wearing no underwear showed no such differences. (Moral of this story? Don't make your pets wear polyester underwear if you want them to have puppies!)

Later, another study found similar effects in humans. Men wearing polyester underwear showed significantly decreased sexual drive compared to men wearing cotton and wool underwear.[26] (Moral of this story? Don't wear polyester underwear or buy polyester underwear for your significant others.) Gynecologist Dr. Hung-Chi Chang also suggested that men wear loose cotton underwear for optimal fertility health, and that women wear cotton underwear to prevent vaginal infections (which are more common when women wear underwear made with less breathable, synthetic fabrics).

Until more specific conclusions can be made about what health effects wearing different textiles can have, we can take a preventative approach by being more selective about our undergarments. If you want to minimize risks of any adverse reactions from what you wear, try to choose organic, natural textiles processed minimally with chemicals for any item of clothing that comes in direct contact with your skin.

Healthier Use, Less Planet Abuse

Not only are the production and disposal of your clothes important; so is the way you use and care for them. A lifecycle analysis on a pair of Levi's 501 jeans found that consumer care and cotton cultivation created the most environmental impact over the jeans' life cycle.[27] More specifically, the study revealed that washing the pair of jeans after wearing it 10 times instead of after wearing it just twice reduced energy use and water intake by 80%![28] You, my reader, have a lot of power in your hands.

To reduce your personal ecological footprint (and also your utilities bill) from caring for your clothes, you can:

- Wash your clothes less often.

- Wash your clothes with cold water instead of hot water.

- If practical, and in a dry and hot climate, hang your clothes up to dry instead of using the dryer.

- Use plant-based, biodegradable laundry detergent instead of petroleum-based detergent.

- If the clothing has an odor, try hanging it up to air it out instead of tossing it right into the washing machine.

Do you ever wonder how your dry-cleaners wash your clothes? Unfortunately, conventional dry-cleaning methods involve a chemical called perchloroethylene (PERC), which is known to cause a variety of adverse health effects. According to the Natural Resources Defense Council (NRDC), exposures to large doses of PERC can affect the central nervous system, liver, and kidneys, and can cause headaches, fatigue, and even mood and behavioral changes.[29] In addition, even chronic exposures to lower levels can impair cognitive and motor functions and cause headaches, vision impairment, and potentially liver damage and adverse kidney effects.

So, what can you do to steer clear of this chemical? Ask your dry cleaners what they use to clean your clothes, even if they advertise themselves as "green" cleaners. The NRDC recommends looking for "Professional Wet Cleaning"[30]—a nontoxic washing method that uses biodegradable detergents and produces no hazardous byproducts—as your best option.

Once you own a piece of clothing, the rest of its environmental impacts depend on *you* and the choices you make. By making more informed decisions on how you can most safely and efficiently care for your clothes, you can be sure to minimize their environmental impacts as well as your personal ecological footprint.

Chapter Summary

Keep in Mind What's Out of Sight

Within any functioning ecosystem, one's waste always goes on to become something of value to another in a continuous, balanced cycle. However, our current waste system is not sustainable, because of the shocking rate at which we throw things out and the problematic types of garbage we create. To address the problems of our garbage mountains and trash vortexes, we need to cherish the things we own more, reduce the amount of stuff we throw out, and prioritize buying 100% **biodegradable** and 100% **indefinitely recyclable** products as much as possible.

Reduce: Less Is More

For a more sustainable future in fashion, we must look for **quality** over the **quantity** of what we buy. Ask yourself questions before you head over to the cashier: Where will this clothing be in 5 or 10 years? Is it durable? Will this purchase aggravate social and environmental issues? What is its impact?

Long-Lasting Materials, Long-Lasting Issues

To address widespread plastic pollution, we need to minimize the amount of clothing we buy made from new, nonbiodegradable materials such as polyester, acrylic, nylon, PVC, and so on. Some relatively healthier alternatives include recycled polyester, recycled nylon, recycled acrylic, and eco-intelligent polyester.

Keep It Simple

To avoid adverse health effects from the chemical residues on your clothing, look for fashion products with simple textile properties. Unless there is explicit information regarding what chemicals were used, avoid clothing labeled "flame retardant," "stain resistant," "odor-free," etc. These usually mean that extra chemicals, likely toxic ones, were used to finish the fabric.

They Persist a While and May Make You Infertile

Some research suggests that wearing polyester underwear may harm fertility health in men, and that wearing polyester fabric can alter normal muscle activity. To avoid potential health effects from the clothes you wear, look for undergarments (or any clothing that comes in direct contact with your skin) made with natural and minimally finished fabrics.

Chapter Summary (Cont'd)

Healthier Use, Less Planet Abuse

A significant part of your clothing's environmental impact depends on how you care for it. Wash your clothes less often, wash with cold water, hang them up to air out odors, and air dry your clothes if possible. Avoid toxic PERC dry cleaning, and look for **professional wet washing** instead.

Chapter 20

Sustain Fashion

The concept of "sustainable fashion" is almost paradoxical. How can fashion—constantly evolving with the ins and outs of the latest trends—achieve sustainability? Unfortunately, there is no clear-cut solution. It is, indeed, a challenge that will require time, drastic changes within the fashion system, and changes in our consumer shopping thought processes. Here are a few tips on how we can adopt healthier mindsets in our fashion choices:

- Choose quality over quantity.

- Choose timeless over trendy.

- Choose slow fashion over fast fashion.

- Choose practical over desirable.

- Choose low-impact materials over high-impact materials.

Now that we have discussed why it is important to *avoid* buying clothing made with virgin, nonbiodegradable fibers (polyester, acrylic, etc.) as much as possible, we also need to know what our healthier options are. After all, we still need to wear clothes, because walking around in public unclothed is generally not considered to be socially acceptable. Plus, shopping for clothes every so often to freshen up our appearances is enjoyable!

When we begin to compare how eco-friendly different textiles are, however, it becomes clear that this comparison is extremely complex. There are so many factors to consider—water usage, human toxicity levels, environmental toxicity levels, biodegradability, energy use, land use, etc.—and it is difficult to determine how we should weigh the relative importance we assign to each of them. In addition, every stage of a product's life cycle must be considered: textile supply, production, retail, use, waste disposal, and transport.[31] This causes discrepancies among different analyses attempting to rank how sustainable various textile choices are. It can be very confusing.

However, as a start, just remember that to truly consider a product as "sustainable," we must think of its impacts in a more holistic manner, judging the importance of multiple factors rather than focusing on any particular one. That said, the quest to a greener future in fashion is no simple task, and any little positive steps taken deserve our support and approval.

New Is Relative

The most environmentally friendly fashion items are those that already exist. Not only do secondhand and vintage clothing have zero impacts from the material sourcing and production phases (because they already exist), but your reuse of them renews their lives and prevents them from ending up in landfills. Many times, you will find clothing or accessories that are in like-new condition in thrift shops or secondhand stores. Plus, most of the time, you will find amazing deals and get more bang for your buck.

Another alternative to buying secondhand is to rent clothing from fashion rental companies (e.g., Rent the Runway), as they try to make as many uses as possible out of every piece of clothing they own. Especially for special occasion outfits—such as costumes or formal attire—that you end up wearing only once, check local thrift shops, rental stores, or reseller platforms such as ThredUp, PoshMark, eBay, Darpdecade, or social media groups for exciting new (but old) finds!

Additionally, you can look for *up-cycled products* or ones made with *up-cycled materials*—that is, old products remade and altered into new products. For example, if an unwanted vintage leather coat is cut up and made into a leather wallet, the wallet is considered "up-cycled." Since little to no new materials are produced, and it recreates value by converting abandoned items into new ones, up-cycling is an artistic, smart, and eco-fashion alternative that deserves more attention.

On the flipside, when it comes time for you to dispose of your clothing, make sure you do so responsibly. You can earn some cash by trying to resell old clothing through companies such as ThredUp or PoshMark, host or attend clothing swaps with your friends and neighbors, or donate it to Goodwill and other charities. If they are not in conditions to be reused, recycle them properly according to your local municipal rules of waste disposal. Even if something may not be of use to you anymore, how wonderful would it be if you can "dispose" of it in a way that can help renew its life?

"Natural" Does not Always Equal "Eco-Friendly"

Although clothes made from plant fibers—one of the two categories of natural fibers—are biodegradable, they are not all considered environmentally friendly. Cotton, for example, is the world's second most damaging agricultural crop.[32] The growing of cotton requires massive amounts of water and pesticide use. While cotton cultivation occupies around 2.5% of the world's agricultural surface, cotton growing alone uses 15.7% of all insecticides and 6.8% of all pesticides.[33] In addition, according to the World Wildlife Fund, it takes a shocking 2,700 liters of water to produce the cotton needed to make one single T-shirt.[34] That's enough water to keep you hydrated for almost three years!

Once one of the largest lakes in the world, the Aral Sea (an inland water basin between Kazakhstan and Uzbekistan) has been drained largely from conventional cotton cultivation, leaving the lake currently at less than 25% of its original size.[35] While cotton is natural and biodegradable, its heavy reliance on water and agrochemicals makes virgin cotton clothes not as green as they may appear.

Some healthier alternatives that address conventional cotton's disadvantages include recycled cotton, naturally rain-fed cotton, and organic cotton. Other relatively more eco-friendly natural fibers from plants include hemp and organic or dew-retted flax (or linen).

Viscose, while biodegradable, is a material considered "synthetic" because it is man-made from wood pulp (typically from beech or eucalyptus trees). While cultivating these trees is considered to be low impact, the manufacturing phase of viscose requires heavy chemical use. The process also emits sulphur, nitrous oxides, carbon disulphide, and hydrogen sulphide into the air and contaminates water from the wastes it generates.[36] Therefore, viscose, while biodegradable, is not really a healthy textile choice because of the amount of air and water pollution its production generates.

More recently, some eco-fashion companies have begun to advertise "bamboo" fabric as a sustainable alternative. However, a lot of fabric made from bamboo is simply bamboo viscose, or viscose made from bamboo pulp. Therefore, it involves the same chemically intensive process as the typical viscose does, and to call it simply bamboo would be "green-washing." If you come upon something made with "bamboo," dig deeper and see if it is merely "bamboo viscose." If so, beware of being green-washed into thinking it is an eco-friendly fabric choice.

Because little management and few pesticides are needed for growing eucalyptus and bamboo, however, improving technology for better ways to process wood pulp seems to be promising. For example, lyocell (or Tencel°), a similar type of fabric made with cellulosic fibers, involves a viscose-like process of manufacturing but recovers almost all of its own wastes. Therefore, lyocell is a more healthful alternative to viscose, and bamboo lyocell is a better choice than bamboo viscose.

The second category of natural textiles includes fabrics made from animal fibers such as wool, cashmere, alpaca, camel, silk, mohair, and so on. While they are all biodegradable, however, much of their environmental impact depends on the conditions the animals were raised in. As with any type of farming, the animals might have been mistreated or raised in unnatural conditions. While it is difficult to know how animals are raised just from looking at a piece of clothing, product descriptions might provide insights into where and how they were raised and can serve as an indication of higher transparency and more responsible practices. For example, labels such as "peace silk" or "wild silk" signify that the silkworms were raised in open forests where no hazardous chemicals were used. Instead of killing them to obtain their silk, as is conventionally done in silk harvesting, peace silk is collected only after the worms have naturally left their chrysalis. In other words, this type of silk is simply made from the silkworms' wastes.

As for wool products, look for certifications that indicate they are organic or pastured, which helps to address problems associated with potential livestock maltreatment and irresponsible waste management. Although wool production may have a high-pollution potential, it still uses three to five times less energy than the production of synthetic fibers such as polyester, nylon, and acrylic.[37] Therefore, so long as the animals are raised healthily and the greasy byproducts from wool processing are managed responsibly, wool (including alpaca, mohair, angora, camel, etc.) is generally considered to be a relatively low-impact fabric option.

The Plight of Hides

Animal pelts make up the last category of biodegradable textiles. However, whether or not to buy leather and fur is extremely controversial, because of a plethora of potentially complex problems.

First, whether or not it is acceptable to wear animal products is a touchy subject. Everyone has his or her own belief regarding this subject, which needs to be respected.

Second, not all pelts are created equal. Two pieces of leather that look exactly the same can have vastly different environmental impacts. For example, do they come from factory-farmed livestock, or from sustainably raised livestock?

Were the animals raised for their skins? Are the hides byproducts of sustainable meat production? Or are they from the wild?

Even pelts from wildlife can vary in their environmental impacts. For example, hides and fur from unmanaged or illegal hunting can endanger species and contribute to biodiversity loss. Meanwhile, hides and fur from strictly regulated hunting that help to alleviate problems with poaching or wildlife population control can even be considered beneficial to ecological health.

Although hunting may seem completely contradictory to conservation, remember that sustainability is about maintaining a *balance* within ecosystems. The World Wildlife Fund, one of the largest international conservation organizations, even supports specific hunting projects around the world—given that they are culturally appropriate, effectively regulated, and have demonstrated environmental and community benefits—in efforts to maintain harmony between humans and nature. As you can see, even putting personal beliefs aside, and depending on where they originate, pelts can still have a wide range of environmental impacts.

The situation gets especially ugly in the manufacturing phase of pelts for fashion. Although some indigenous populations today and humans since the earliest of times have made clothing from pelts without any industrialized chemicals, the majority of leather and fur sold today are heavily processed and treated with toxic chemicals and dyes. Therefore, because of the high-pollution potential of animal pelts produced for fashion, they are generally considered not to be eco-friendly, whether or not they come from sustainable sources.

What about faux fur and the so-called "vegan leather"? Well, faux fur is often made out of a mix of nonbiodegradable, petrochemical-based materials (often with high pollution potentials). And, even though some vegan leather is made of natural cork or recycled plastics, many of these products are made with polyvinyl chloride (PVC), another petroleum-based material. While PVC is "cruelty-free," it is an extremely toxic material that does not break down in nature and releases hazardous chemicals when incinerated. This makes PVC almost impossible to dispose of without harming the environment and threatening our health.

The manufacturing of PVC also produces an extremely toxic byproduct called *dioxins*, a chemical that can bioaccumulate in the food chain, cause reproductive and developmental problems, damage the immune system, and cause cancer.[38] Unfortunately, these persisting pollutants have been found all over the world and have already come back to us in our own food sources: meat, dairy products, fish, and shellfish.[39] So, are they truly "cruelty-free?"

With improving technology, we can only hope that healthier fur and leather options become feasible for us in the future. At the current moment, however, unless you are given information regarding where a pelt originated from and how it was dyed and treated (i.e., through certifications or voluntary information), it may be safest to just stick to secondhand, recycled, or up-cycled faux and real pelts.

A Biodiverse Wardrobe, A Biodiverse Planet

The key to sustainable fashion, like the key to a sustainable diet, is *diversity*. There is no one perfect fabric choice out there, because sustainability depends on *balancing* our resources.

For example, organic hemp is one of our most eco-friendly fabric options right now. But if everyone were to buy only organic hemp clothing, too much pressure would be exerted on that one resource. This would result in a loss of biodiversity, hence the deterioration of our planet's overall health.

When the herders in Mongolia increased their goat population to meet higher demand for cashmere, the once-thriving pastures began to degrade, leading to desertification of their lands. The pastures were simply unable to sustain the increasing pressures from the growing goat population. While clothing made from alpaca fibers has recently been touted as being eco-friendly, it won't be so in another decade if demands for it continue to grow exponentially.

Therefore, instead of searching for one perfect fabric type, we need to constantly diversify our options and support the production of inventive new fibers. For example, some small-scale manufacturers have ventured into turning banana peels or pineapple leaves, which would otherwise be thrown away, into textiles. Others are using technology to find novel ways to turn trash, such as plastic bottles and even old fire hoses, into usable fabrics.

Table 20-1 on the next page summarizes which common fabric types you should minimize buying (whether shopping for fashion products, home furnishings, or other products) while providing some healthier alternatives to those fabrics.

Keep in mind that these are my personal, qualitative suggestions and that the comparison is relative, as no fabric type is all good or all bad. Note also that I strongly emphasize avoiding new, nonbiodegradable fabrics and ones with high pollution potentials, because, while we can continually improve energy and water efficiency, it is less plausible to conduct global cleanups of microplastic pollution and widespread chemical contamination.

Table 20-1. A Shopping Guide for Healthier Textile Choices

Category	Minimize...	Some healthier alternatives
Synthetic fabrics	Polyester, nylon, acrylic, PVC leather, faux fur made with a mix of synthetic materials	Recycled polyester, recycled nylon, recycled acrylic, recycled or up-cycled fabrics, and Eco-Intelligent® Polyester (a type of nontoxic polyester by Victor Innovatex that is indefinitely recyclable)
Synthetic fabrics from natural origins	Viscose, bamboo viscose	Lyocell (or Tencel® by Lenzing), bamboo lyocell, and recycled or up-cycled fabrics
Natural fabrics from plant fibers	Cotton	Organic cotton, rain-fed cotton, hemp, organic flax, dew-retted flax, and recycled or up-cycled fabrics
Natural fabrics from animal fibers	Conventional silk, cheap and mass-produced animal fibers from irresponsible herding or factory farms	Organic wool, recycled animal fibers, peace or wild silk, fibers from responsibly raised alpaca, mohair, sheep, and other animals, and up-cycled fabrics
Pelts	Leather, fur, shearling	Recycled leather, recycled animal fur, low-impact pelts, and up-cycled or secondhand pelts

As Kate Fletcher, author of *Sustainable Fashion and Textiles,* noted, we need to develop a portfolio of many diverse, sustainable textiles.[40] Some may be more water intensive; others will be more energy intensive. However, these relatively healthier, more mindful options altogether will help reduce the amount of non-biodegradable trash we generate, decrease overall environmental impacts from the fashion industry, and improve the working conditions for everyone involved in the supply chain.

Chapter Summary

New Is Relative

The most environmentally friendly fashion items are the ones that already exist (i.e., vintage, used, secondhand, or up-cycled products), because they technically have zero impacts from their material sourcing and production phases. Plus, your choosing to buy these items will renew their lives by keeping them out of landfills!

"Natural" Doesn't Always Equal "Eco-Friendly"

Not all natural materials are created equal. For example, cotton is extremely water- and pesticide-intensive, and viscose, a synthetic textile made from tree pulp, has a high pollution potential. Currently, some of your relatively more environmentally friendly fabric options include organic or rain-fed cotton, hemp, organic linen, lyocell (or bamboo lyocell), peace silk, and other types of animal fibers such as alpaca and wool (if the animals were raised naturally with minimal environmental impact).

The Plight of Hides

Because the manufacturing of pelts today uses a lot of toxic chemicals, most commercially sold leather and fur products are not considered to be very healthy. Unless you personally know where a pelt originated from and how it was processed and dyed (i.e., with certifications or other voluntary information), your healthiest choice is just to buy recycled, up-cycled, or secondhand leather or fur products.

A Biodiverse Wardrobe, A Biodiverse Planet

The future for a more sustainable fashion system is not about finding one perfect material. Exerting too much pressure on any one type of resource can lead to biodiversity loss and land degradation. Instead, we need to diversify our relatively more eco-friendly material choices and support technology for new, inventive fibers (e.g., fibers made from banana peels, pineapple leaves, recycled plastic bottles, etc.).

Chapter 21

Look Good Doing Good

A recurring motif in this book is balance—but a balance between sometimes seemingly opposing concepts: caring for oneself versus being selfless; indulging in the current moment versus maintaining long-term health; embracing consumerism versus working toward sustainability. These are just some of the struggles many of us face in our daily lives. However, there is no need for an ultimatum, and we don't always have to choose one or the other.

When we begin to see that we impact others as much as they impact us, it becomes clear that sometimes being selfless is the best way to care for ourselves. When we begin to see how our bodies and our planet's ecosystems function and interact with one another, we will also fathom the possibility of enjoying life right now while nourishing our minds, bodies, and environment. And finally, when we become more informed consumers, we will better understand how to make meaningful purchases that can help to mitigate the social and environmental problems currently aggravated by our consumer choices.

A Healthy Shopping Mindset

As more and more brands begin to appeal to the health-conscious consumer, *green-washing* is also becoming more common. Many brands market themselves as "ethical" or "sustainable," but what is their basis for determining this? Do they call themselves eco-friendly just because their products are cruelty-free? What if the manufacturing of their products produces byproducts toxic to wildlife? Are these companies "ethical" just because their workers get paid fair wages? But what if these very same workers are forced to work with large quantities of toxic chemicals every day?

There are so many questions we need to begin asking. For now, however, to avoid being green-washed, we need to look past a product's fluffy marketing statements when we shop. Phrases such as "all natural" or "sustainable" are used everywhere and have almost become trite. Look past these unregulated labels and check for the more objective details (e.g., material composition, certifications, etc.). Alden Wicker, eco-lifestyle advocate and founder of Eco-Cult, noted that responsible companies should be open and transparent about the who, what, and why of their clothing rather than just projecting glossy images. If you can't find any additional corporate social responsibility information from a brand that calls itself "sustainable" or "ethical," you have good reason to question whether it truly lives up to its proclaimed standards.

Of course, working toward a healthier fashion industry will take time, for companies must face so many challenges when trying to develop products that meet their visions and are profitable while still taking human and ecosystem health concerns into consideration. This also makes it difficult for us as consumers to shop responsibly 100% of the time. Sometimes, you simply do not have that option. For example, if there is a unique shirt made with virgin polyester that you cannot live without, do not feel guilty for buying it. Given the limited eco-friendly, high-quality, and well-made options we currently have, few are capable of making perfectly sustainable fashion choices 100% of the time. However, keep in mind that, with every question you raise, and with every thoughtful purchasing decision you make, you are helping to push the industry in a healthier direction.

Consumerism Meets Sustainability

As discussed in Part IV, "Beautify," responsible brands value people, planet, and profit (the three *Ps*). First, they care for their workers' and consumers' health. Therefore, they strive toward production processes that minimize the use of agrochemicals, toxic dyes, and toxic chemical finishes.

Many companies that export manufacturing to developing countries also use their power for good by pushing for social changes within their workers' communities. Some help fight for gender equality, some push for sustainable development, and some empower underprivileged families to run their own businesses. For example, People Tree makes its core mission to not only ensure fair trade for all of its sourced products, but also help people in the marginalized communities they work with to escape poverty, strengthen their communities, and promote environmental sustainability. By taking on such voluntary yet transformative initiatives, companies like these are making a statement that they want to be around for good—both ethics-wise and time-wise.

Responsible companies also care for our planet's health. Therefore, they minimize their environmental impacts by cutting down on the production of new, nonbiodegradable products, finding new sources of eco-friendly raw materials, properly handling their wastes, making sure they know the origins of all of their materials, and so on. Patagonia, for example, does an incredible job at using innovative, eco-conscious materials for their large range of outdoor gears. United by Blue, another outdoor apparel brand using its power for good, not only produces environmentally conscious products but also pledges to remove one pound of trash from our waterways for every product sold.

Finally—perhaps needless to say—sustainable brands need to profit so they can continue to operate sustainably. Therefore, they communicate their responsible practices by being more transparent about the stories behind their products. Zady, an extremely influential eco-lifestyle brand, sets an amazing example of how a responsible company should operate. The brand embraces transparency and narrates the stories of their products' entire production processes from start to finish, as if they all really mattered—because they do. After all, every part of a product's life cycle is a story worth knowing.

To help validate claims made by brands, you can also look for third-party labels or certifications. Here are some of the most common ones in the fashion industry, as well as what they signify (see Table 21-2).

Table 21-1. Common Labels in the Fashion Industry

Label	Significance
B Corp	This is a more general certification given to companies that meet rigorous standards of social and environmental performance, accountability, and transparency.
Ecolabel by the European Union	This certification denotes products with reduced environmental impacts throughout their life cycle.
Fair Trade	The Fair Trade label guarantees that farmers and workers involved in the production process were compensated justly for their work. While it is more of a validation of ethical practices, the nonprofit also promotes sustainable agriculture.
GCC Brandmark	The GCC brand mark by Eco Age is a validation for individual products or fashion collections that meet rigorous social, ethical, and environmental standards.
Global Organic Textile Standard (GOTS)	Certified textiles contain at least 70% of organic fibers, and all chemicals used must meet strict criteria. Proper wastewater treatments are also mandatory.
Made-By	This label assures that a brand operates responsibly with respect to people and the planet.

Table 21-1. Common Labels in the Fashion Industry Cont'd

Label	Significance
Oeko-Tex® Standard 100	This certification ensures that the tested yarns and textiles do not contain illegal substances, regulated harmful substances, or known harmful but unregulated chemicals.
PETA-Approved Vegan	This is a symbol by People for the Ethical Treatment of Animals (PETA) used by companies that make vegan and animal-friendly clothing and accessories.
USDA Organic	The USDA certification is made for organic agricultural practices (like Ecocert, Soil Association, etc.). Therefore, a USDA organic certification for a cotton shirt ensures that the cotton was grown organically, but does not guarantee that the shirt is free of toxic finishes.
World Fair Trade Organization (WFTO)	The WFTO is a fair trade certification that ensures responsible practices across the supply chain and supports small producers and their communities.

Finally, to sum up the past few chapters, here are some personal tips I give to people who want to pick out environmentally conscious, thoughtfully made fashion products (or any other general consumer products):

- Look at the material composition of the product.

- Look for certifications and labels.

- Look for descriptions regarding where, how and by whom the product was made, and with what materials, dyes, and chemicals.

- If a product has broad marketing labels such as "eco-friendly" with no supporting evidence whatsoever, ask questions and contact the product's brand representative for more information.

- Learn more about the brand that made the product by visiting its social media pages and official website.

When you come to realize that every product has its own story, shopping becomes much more meaningful than just empty purchases of some flattering shirt or some trendy scarf. By understanding the histories of our daily consumer products, we can connect to a world greater than ourselves through our shopping experiences. By collectively asking questions, challenging the current system, and supporting responsible companies, we can shop our way together to a better, healthier world.

Chapter Summary

A Healthy Shopping Mindset

To avoid being deceived by misleading marketing statements, look past vague, unsubstantiated labels such as "sustainable" or "ethical." Instead, seek out your more objective indicators of the whos, whats, whens, wheres, whys, and hows behind the product. Although it is ideal to buy only responsible products, this is often not possible, given the limited choices we currently have. However, with every thoughtful purchase you make, you are helping to push the industry in a healthier direction.

Consumerism Meets Sustainability

Responsible companies value people, planet, and profit—the three Ps. Check for certifications and information provided on their social media pages or official websites, and ask their brand representative questions about their practices. When you see that all consumer products have rich histories awaiting your discovery, your shopping experience can become so much more meaningful. It will not only engage your mind and heart in the process, but also connect you to a world greater than yourself.

Chapter 22

Detox Your Home

There is no place like home—the warm, memory-filled dwelling you grew up in, the place you return to at the end of a long day, and the sanctuary that rejuvenates you before you go back to face the outside world. Of course, you want this place to be safe and peaceful—a place that helps you de-stress and unwind from the fast-paced modern world.

You spray some air freshener to freshen up the air in your home, and then you calmly take a deep breath to inhale the lavender, lemon-infused scent. But beware: You are probably also taking in some volatile organic compounds (VOCs)—substances that can irritate your eyes, nose, and throat, damage your central nervous system and other organs, and might even be carcinogenic.[41,42]

Unfortunately, VOCs come not only from typical air fresheners, but also from paints and building supplies, toilet deodorizers, mothballs, other aerosol spray products (e.g., hairspray, aerosol sunscreen), chlorine bleach, detergent, cheap candles, and dry-cleaning chemical residues. Indoor air pollution can also come from dust (some is shed from garment fibers); lead from wall paint or drinking water; formaldehyde from pressed wood products, combustion sources, or even clothing; and smoke from residential wood, cheap candles, or incense burning, among many, many others.

According to the World Health Organization, 3.8 million premature deaths every year from noncommunicable diseases such as stroke, chronic obstructive pulmonary diseases, and lung cancer can be attributed to exposure to household air pollution.[43] Can your safe haven be slowly damaging your health?

Invisible Threats

Many of us overlook the problem of air pollution by thinking it is only a problem for the outdoors. However, the air inside your office and home can also be polluted by various sources: household products, pesticides, materials used in the building, etc. According to the US Consumer Product Safety Commission (CPSC), indoor air can be more seriously polluted than outdoor air, even in the most industrialized cities.[44] Since most of us spend a lot of our time indoors, we need to shop mindfully also for our home products: cleaning supplies, furniture, home decor, wall paint, etc.

To help you get started, here is a list of tips to help you reduce indoor air pollution in your home:[45,46]

Home Habits

- Do not smoke inside.

- Avoid burning wood, cheap and scented candles, and incense indoors.

- Use high-quality soy or beeswax-based candles over cheap ones made with paraffin wax.

- Cover your trash, and do not leave food out in the open.

- Ventilate your home often.

Home Care

- Avoid aerosol spray cans for air fresheners and household cleaners.

- Avoid pesticides within your home, and address the source of the problem instead (i.e., not leaving food out).

- Look for simple, biodegradable household cleaning products that disclose all ingredients used.

- Look for household cleaning products labeled "no fragrance."

- Toss out expired or unneeded chemicals and products safely.

- Vacuum and dust your home frequently.

- Get your tap water tested for lead and other chemical pollutants. While most city water is tested and is free of contaminants, pollutants can enter your tap water from old pipes or household plumbing.

Home Furnishing

- Choose non-PVC wall paint and floor finishes.

- Choose solid wood over pressed wood.

- Choose formaldehyde-free insulation and furnishing materials when re-modeling your home.

- Ventilate your home well when refurbishing.

To effectively detox your home, try to be more careful about what home products you buy. This means looking past the soothing appearances of the next paint color you want for your walls, the relaxing scents of your air deodorizers and household cleaners, and the stylish look of the new rug you want for your bedroom. Instead, ask the same questions you would ask when shopping for your self-care and fashion products, for example:

- Is the brand transparent about what their products are made of?

- Does the brand care about people and our planet's health?

- Are there any certifications, such as the "Safer Choice Label" recently developed by the US EPA, that can affirm their safety record?

To make shopping for healthy cleaning products easier, you can apply the less-is-more principle as well. Do you really need a bathtub cleaner, a countertop cleaner, a sink cleaner, and an oven cleaner? Instead, you can often find all-purpose cleaners made with simple biodegradable, plant-based ingredients.

Since companies are not required to list their ingredients, those that openly tell you what their products comprise are usually your most trusted options. For example, Mrs. Meyer's and Method are household supply brands that do an incredible job of disclosing every ingredient used in their products while also informing consumers of each ingredient's function and properties.

After checking the ingredient list, look out for certifications indicating that the product is biodegradable and made without petroleum-based chemicals. Additionally, if the products have warning labels such as "DANGER" or "POISON," you probably do not want them lurking in your house.

As the CPSC noted, source control is the most effective solution to indoor air pollution.[47] Therefore, the best way to detox your home is to prevent polluting sources from entering it in the first place and eliminating potentially hazardous wastes from sitting around in your house. In other words, practice healthier home-care habits, shop mindfully for your self-care, fashion, and home products, simplify the number of household products you use, and find ones with simple, clearly labeled ingredient lists. Otherwise, try the following home remedies that have been tested as safe and effective by the Toxics Use Reduction Institute Laboratory so you won't have to worry about any potential unknown pollutants.[48] (See Table 22-1.)

Table 22-1. Home Remedies for Household Cleaning[49]

Surface to be cleaned	Home remedy
All-purpose cleaner	Dissolve 4 tablespoons of baking soda in 1 qt. warm water. Wipe and scrub to clean. No rinsing needed.
All-purpose cleaner	Add 2 tablespoons borax, 1/4 cup lemon juice, and 2 cups hot water into a spray bottle. Spray and wipe to clean.
Metal surfaces such as the oven	Mix 2 tablespoons of vegetable oil soap, 2 table-spoons of borax, and 6 oz. warm water in a spray bottle. Spray on surface and use an abrasive pad for extra cleaning. Leave on for 20 minutes and wipe away.
Aluminum and copper surfaces like those for pots and pans	Soak in 50:50 water and vinegar mixture for at least 15 minutes (or overnight) and rinse.
Bathroom surfaces such as ceramic, plastic, and metal	Mix 1/4 cup vinegar in one gallon of water to wipe or scrub.
Window surfaces with glass and chrome	Mix 50:50 vinegar and water to wipe clean.

Lower Environmental Impact, Lower Utility Bills

To truly turn your home into an environmentally conscious home, you must also minimize your energy and water use and the amount of waste you generate. The upside of this mindset is that it will be better for the environment, your health, and your savings account.

For example, you can save electricity by taking full advantage of natural daylight and going to sleep when it becomes dark outside. As we discussed in chapter 8, "Sleep Productively," slowly dimming your lights to mimic the gradual fading of natural daylight as it nears your bedtime can help you to sleep better. In addition, waking up to natural daylight can also help you wake up more easily in the morning. So, turn down your lights as the evening progresses, and open up all of your curtains during the day to take advantage of natural sunlight.

Another way to reduce your energy usage is to lessen your use of air conditioners and heaters. Do you ever find 60 degrees Fahrenheit (15.6 degrees Celsius) to be cold when summer first transitions into autumn, but hot when winter transitions into spring? This is because our bodies are capable of adjusting to varying temperatures to a certain extent, which means there is no one perfect room temperature you must maintain in your home.

Instead, be mindful of your body. Are you really burning up and need some cold air (i.e., you must use your air conditioner), or will it suffice to open the window or turn on the fan to gain a little ventilation? Are you really freezing, or can you just throw on another sweater and a pair of socks? Our bodies are extremely complex, and thermal regulation is one of their natural functions. So, mind your body and give it a few minutes to adjust to a new environment before deciding you need to turn on the air conditioning or heater.

In addition to minimizing your use of lights, AC, and heaters, here are some other tips on how to save electricity:

- Turn off your electronics when you are not using them. They can still use up to 60% of power when on "standby."

- Unplug your chargers from their sockets when not in use.

- Use energy-efficient light bulbs, such as LED lighting.

- Wash your clothes with cold water instead of hot water.

- Air-dry your clothes instead of using the dryer, if possible.

- Shower with warm, not hot, water (which, as discussed in Chapter 17, is also healthier for your skin).

- Do not leave your refrigerator doors open.

- If you are refurnishing your home, install better insulation into your walls so they will keep your home cooler in the summer and warmer in the winter.

Freshwater conservation is something most of us know is important, but why should we be more mindful about the amount of water we use right now? Unfortunately, at our current rate of water usage, the World Health Organization estimates that by 2025, half of our world's population will be living in water-stressed areas.[50] This means that our current rate of usage is *not* sustainable. And why is this alarming? Clean water is one of the basic survival necessities for *all* living species on our planet. Therefore, contaminating our water supply and depleting our freshwater sources will increase global stress and conflict, threaten public welfare, drive many living species to the point of endangerment or even extinction, and, at worst, even lead to the downfall of you, me, and our entire planet!

As the EPA stated, "It takes many years and it is very costly to remove contamination affecting water supplies. Often the damage is *irreparable,* and the water resource can never be used as a drinking water source again."[51] Because it is much easier and less costly to prevent pollution in the first place than to contaminate our natural environment and then try to clean up afterward, we will all benefit by taking a more preventative approach to water conservation. To do so, we need to support sustainable agriculture that minimizes the use of agrochemicals; buy self-care products, fashion pieces, home-cleaning supplies, and other products made minimally with toxic materials and substances; and minimize the amount of water we each use for all purposes other than drinking.

Here are some simple water conservation tips:

- Install low-flow faucet aerators on all of your faucets. This is the easiest, most effortless way to save water.

- Run the dishwasher and washing machine only when they are full.

- Wash your clothes less often.

- Do not let the water run when you're not using it.

- Keep showers to five minutes or less. As dermatologist Sandra T. Yeh suggested in Chapter 17, this is also a healthier way to maintain your skin's natural protective barrier.

Finally, you can make your home more environmentally oriented by reducing the amount of waste you generate. If the zero-waste lifestyle (i.e., a lifestyle that does not produce garbage intended for the landfills) has already been proven possible by dedicated model citizens such as Bea Johnson, a wife and mother of two residing in California, as well as Lauren Singer, a recent graduate living in New York, I am sure you will have no problem cutting down on the quantity of waste you generate by following these tips:

- Bring your own reusable containers or eating utensils for take-out food.

- Cut down on the amount of packaged food you buy (this will encourage you to eat healthier as well).

- Use reusable water bottles.

- Use reusable shopping bags.

- Buy products with minimal packaging.

- Buy products in bulk.

- Focus on quality over quantity in everything you buy.

Alternatively, just keep Bea Johnson's five R's in mind: *Refuse, Reduce, Reuse, Recycle,* and *Rot* (and only in that order).

When it comes time to throw out whatever trash you still have left, however, make sure you do so thoughtfully. This means following the garbage and recycling rules of your local community, reselling or donating anything that is still in good and working condition, and properly disposing of hazardous waste.

For example, refrain from pouring old cleaning supplies that may contain toxic chemicals down the drain, and separate your old electronic goods and used batteries from the rest of your trash. Because electrical equipment and consumer electronics contain heavy metals and other materials that are extremely toxic to human health and the environment, they need to be disposed of in special facilities. Sometimes you can recycle old electronics by returning them to the stores you bought them from. Otherwise, just separate your hazardous waste from the rest of your trash when you discard it.

An Eco-Sanctuary

To transform your home into a healthy and relaxing sanctuary, let us return to the concept of *biophilia*, the theory backed by evidence that we have an innate need to affiliate with nature and can obtain health benefits from simple exposures to natural landscapes. If you are not going to be spending the majority of your time outdoors, maybe you can obtain similar benefits by inviting the outdoors in.

Why not recreate the soothing experience of being enveloped by nature inside of your home? For example, you can accessorize your interiors with indoor plants. Although they may not be able to get rid of all your indoor air pollutants, they can help to naturally freshen up your air! When shopping for plants, look for species endemic to your region to help preserve your local species diversity and prevent problems with *invasive species*, which are nonnative animals, plants, or pathogens to an ecosystem that are likely to cause harm if introduced. If the environmental conditions are ideal for any newly introduced, nonnative species, they can become problematic, as the lack of predator or competitor species will allow them to spread and take over native landscapes. In other words, they can disrupt the balance within your local ecosystem and contribute to habitat degradation, biodiversity loss of native species, crop damage, and potential diseases in humans and livestock. So, when possible, choose regional plant varieties over exotic ones, and refrain from bringing home exotic seeds from abroad.

To simulate nature in your home in ways other than bringing in plants, you can decorate your indoor space with other elements from nature. For example, you can use wooden furniture or wooden home accessories for interior decor, or hang paintings or photographs reminiscent of nature. When buying forest products such as paper, notebooks, wooden furniture, or wooden accessories, look for the Forest Stewardship Council (FSC) certification to ensure the material was harvested from sustainably managed forests. Alternatively, look for products made with reclaimed wood or post-consumer recycled materials. To avoid chemical pollutants such as formaldehyde from entering your house, choose minimally-finished wooden products made with solid wood over pressed wood, an engineered material made from artificially bonding wood shavings together. This way, you will be inviting the outdoors in with minimal environmental and health impacts.

Once you have detoxified your home, reduced the environmental impacts of your house, and styled your personal space with elements from nature, you will have built for yourself an eco-sanctuary you can return to every night for true rejuvenation and worry-free relaxation.

Chapter Summary

Invisible Threats

Indoor air pollution is an often-overlooked health threat many home products and cleaning supplies contribute to. To detox your home, look beyond the appearances of the products and supplies you bring into the house and see what materials or ingredients they are made of. Ask the same questions you would ask before buying new fashion or self-care products, e.g.: Does the company care about people and our planet? Is it transparent about its manufacturing process? What chemicals or ingredients are used?

Lower Environmental Impact, Lower Utility Bills

To transform your home into an environmentally conscious home, you will have to be more mindful of how much energy and water you use and how much trash you generate. Cutting down on all of these will be beneficial to your health, our planet's health, and your savings account. Think efficiency, savings, and quality over quantity.

An Eco-Sanctuary

As discussed in Part I, "Smile," we can potentially obtain health benefits simply by getting in touch with nature. To turn your home into an eco-sanctuary you can feel safe and relaxed in, detox your home, lower its environmental impact, and style your interiors with indoor plants and other elements of nature.

Part References

1   Gardetti, M. A., & Muthu, S. S. (2015). *Handbook of sustainable luxury textiles and fashion* (Vol. 1). Singapore: Springer.

2   Kant, R. (2012). Textile dyeing industry: An environmental hazard. *Natural Science, 04*(01), 22-26.

3   Nimbalker, G., Mawson, J., Cremen, C., Wrinkle, H., & Eriksson, E. (2015). *The Australian fashion report 2015* (Rep.). Baptist World Aid Australia. Retrieved from http://www.baptistworldaid.org.au/assets/Be-Fair-Section/FashionReport.pdf

4   Derraik, J. G. (2002). The pollution of the marine environment by plastic debris: A review. *Marine Pollution Bulletin, 44*(9), 842-852.

5   Laist, D. W. (1997). Impacts of marine debris: Entanglement of marine life in marine debris including a comprehensive list of species with entanglement and ingestion records. *Springer Series on Environmental Management Marine Debris*, 99-139.

6   Rochman, C. M., Tahir, A., Williams, S. L., Baxa, D. V., Lam, R., Miller, J. T., . . . Teh, S. J. (2015). Anthropogenic debris in seafood: Plastic debris and fibers from textiles in fish and bivalves sold for human consumption. *Scientific Reports, 5*, 14340.

7   Rochman, C. M., Hoh, E., Kurobe, T., & Teh, S. J. (2013). Ingested plastic transfers hazardous chemicals to fish and induces hepatic stress. *Scientific Reports, 3*, 3263.

8   Rochman, C. M., Tahir, A., Williams, S. L., Baxa, D. V., Lam, R., Miller, J. T., . . . Teh, S. J. (2015). Anthropogenic debris in seafood: Plastic debris and fibers from textiles in fish and bivalves sold for human consumption. *Scientific Reports, 5*, 14340.

9   As cited in Claudio, L. (2007). Waste couture: Environmental impact of the clothing industry. *Environmental Health Perspectives, 115*(9), A449-A454.

10 McDonough, W., & Braungart, M. (2002). *Cradle to cradle: Remaking the way we make things*. New York: North Point Press.

11 Claudio, L. (2007). Waste couture: Environmental impact of the clothing industry. *Environmental Health Perspectives, 115*(9), A449-A454.

12 Browne, M. A., Crump, P., Niven, S. J., Teuten, E., Tonkin, A., Galloway, T., & Thompson, R. (2011). Accumulation of microplastics on shorelines

worldwide: Sources and sinks. *Environmental Science & Technology, 45*(21), 9175-9179.

13   Browne, M. A., Crump, P., Niven, S. J., Teuten, E., Tonkin, A., Galloway, T., & Thompson, R. (2011). Accumulation of microplastics on shorelines worldwide: Sources and sinks. *Environmental Science & Technology, 45*(21), 9175-9179.

14   Engler, R. E. (2012). The Complex interaction between marine debris and toxic chemicals in the ocean. *Environmental Science & Technology, 46*(22), 12302-12315.

15   Seltenrich, N. (2015). New link in the food chain? Marine plastic pollution and seafood safety. *Environmental Health Perspectives, 123*(2), A34-A41.

16   Shim, W. J., & Thompson, R. C. (2015). Microplastics in the ocean. *Archives of Environmental Contamination and Toxicology, 69*(3), 265-268.

17   Kant, R. (2012). Textile dyeing industry: An environmental hazard. *Natural Science, 04*(01), 22-26.

18   Brigden, K., Hetherington, S., Weng, M., Santillo, D., & Johnston, P. (2014). *Hazardous chemicals in branded luxury textile products on sale during 2013* (Rep.). Greenpeace Research Laboratories. Retrieved from http://www.greenpeace.org/international/Global/international/publications /toxics/2014/Technical-Report-01-2014.pdf

19   Brigden, K., Hetherington, S., Weng, M., Santillo, D., & Johnston, P. (2014). *Hazardous chemicals in branded luxury textile products on sale during 2013* (Rep.). Greenpeace Research Laboratories. Retrieved from http://www.greenpeace.org/international/Global/international/publications /toxics/2014/Technical-Report-01-2014.pdf

20   As cited in Clement, A. M. & Clement, B. R. (2011). *Killer clothes: How seemingly innocent clothing choices endanger your health—and how to pro-tect yourself!* Summertown, Tenn.: Hippocrates Publications, p74.

21   As cited in Clement, A. M. & Clement, B. R. (2011). *Killer clothes: How seemingly innocent clothing choices endanger your health—and how to pro-tect yourself!* Summertown, Tenn.: Hippocrates Publications, p69.

22   Lazarov, A. (2004). Textile dermatitis in patients with contact sensitization in Israel: A 4-year prospective study. *Journal of the European Academy of Dermatology and Venereology, 18*(5), 531-537.

23   Zimniewska, M., Huber, J., Krucinska, I., Torlinska, T., & Kozlowski, R. (2002). The influence of clothes made from natural and synthetic fibres on the activity of the motor units in selected muscles in the forearm. *Fibres and Textiles in Eastern Europe*, 55-59.

24 Zimniewska, M., & Krucińska, I. (2010). The effect of raw material composition of clothes on selected physiological parameters of human organism. *Journal of the Textile Institute, 101*(2), 154-164.

25 Shafik, A. (1993). Effect of different types of textile fabric on spermatogenesis: An experimental study. *Urological Research, 21*(5), 367-370.

26 Shafik, A. (1996). Effect of different types of textiles on male sexual activity. *Systems Biology in Reproductive Medicine, 37*(2), 111-115.

27 Levi Strauss & Co. (2015). *The life cycle of a jean: Understanding the environmental impact of a pair of Levi 501 Jeans* (Rep.). Retrieved from http://levistrauss.com/wp-content/uploads/2015/03/Full-LCA-Results-Deck-FINAL.pdf

28 Levi Strauss & Co. (2015). *The life cycle of a jean: Understanding the environmental impact of a pair of Levi 501 Jeans* (Rep.). Retrieved from http://levistrauss.com/wp-content/uploads/2015/03/Full-LCA-Results-Deck-FINAL.pdf

29 Natural Resources Defense Council. (2011a). *How to care for the planet and your health while also caring for your clothes.* Retrieved from http://www.nrdc.org/living/stuff/dry-cleaning.asp

30 Natural Resources Defense Council. (2011a). *How to care for the planet and your health while also caring for your clothes.* Retrieved from http://www.nrdc.org/living/stuff/dry-cleaning.asp

31 Rinaldi, F. R., & Testa, S. (2014). *The responsible fashion company: Integrating ethics and aesthetics in the supply chain.* Sheffield: Greenleaf Publishing, p70.

32 Kant, R. (2012). Textile dyeing industry: An environmental hazard. *Natural Science, 04*(01), 22-26.

33 Styles, R. (2014). *Ecologist guide to fashion.* Lewes: The Ivy Press.

34 World Wildlife Fund. (2013, January 16). *The impact of a cotton T-shirt.* Retrieved from http://www.worldwildlife.org/stories/the-impact-of-a-cotton-t-shirt

35 Allwood, J. M., Laursen, S. E., De Rodríguez, C. M., & Bocken, N. M. (2006). *Well dressed?: The present and future sustainability of clothing and textiles in the United Kingdom.* Cambridge: University of Cambridge, Institute of Manufacturing.

36 Fletcher, K. (2008). *Sustainable fashion and textiles: Design journeys.* London: Earthscan, p19.

37 Fletcher, K. (2008). *Sustainable fashion and textiles: Design journeys.* London: Earthscan, p15.

38 World Health Organization. (2014, June). *Dioxins and their effects on human health*. Retrieved from
http://www.who.int/mediacentre/factsheets/fs225/en/

39 World Health Organization. (2014, June). *Dioxins and their effects on human health*. Retrieved from
http://www.who.int/mediacentre/factsheets/fs225/en/

40 Fletcher, K. (2008). *Sustainable fashion and textiles: Design journeys*. London: Earthscan, p43.

41 Mølhave, L., Bach, B., & Pedersen, O. (1986). Human reactions to low concentrations of volatile organic compounds. *Environment International, 12*(1-4), 167-175.

42 United States Environmental Protection Agency. (n.d.b). *Volatile organic compounds' impact on indoor air quality*. Retrieved from
http://www.epa.gov/indoor-air-quality-iaq/volatile-organic-compounds-impact-indoor-air-quality#Health_Effects

43 World Health Organization. (2014). *Household air pollution and health*. Retrieved from http://www.who.int/mediacentre/factsheets/fs292/en/

44 Consumer Product Safety Commission. (n.d.). *The inside story: A guide to indoor air quality*. Retrieved from http://www.cpsc.gov/en/Safety-Education/Safety-Guides/Home/The-Inside-Story-A-Guide-to-Indoor-Air-Quality/

45 American Lung Association. *52 Proven Stress Reducers (n.d.)*: n. pag. *Freedom From Smoking Online*. American Lung Association. Retrieved from
http://www.ffsonline.org/assets/handouts/module-5/52-proven-stress-reducers.pdf

46 Toxics Use Reduction Institute. (2011). *Ten tips to improve indoor air quality*. Tip Sheet Series. Turi: TURI Publications. TURI Toxics Use Reduction Institute. Retrieved from
http://www.turi.org/TURI_Publications/Tip_Sheet_Series/Ten_Tips_to_Improve_Indoor_Air_Quality

47 Consumer Product Safety Commission. (n.d.). *The inside story: A guide to indoor air quality*. Retrieved from http://www.cpsc.gov/en/Safety-Education/Safety-Guides/Home/The-Inside-Story-A-Guide-to-Indoor-Air-Quality/

48 Toxics Use Reduction Institute Laboratory. (2013). *Twelve home cleaning recipes*. Retrieved from
http://www.turi.org/TURI_Publications/Tip_Sheet_Series/Twelve_Home_Cleaning_Recipes

49 Homemade remedies for cleaning by the Toxics Use Reduction Institute Laboratory. (2013). *Twelve home cleaning recipes*. Retrieved from http://www.turi.org/TURI_Publications/Tip_Sheet_Series/Twelve_Home_Cleaning_Recipes

50 World Health Organization. (2015, June). *Drinking-water*. Retrieved from http://www.who.int/mediacentre/factsheets/fs391/en/

51 United States Environmental Protection Agency. (n.d.a). *Preventing contamination of drinking water resources*. Retrieved from http://www3.epa.gov/region1/eco/drinkwater/prevent_contamination.html

PART VI

TRANSFORM

*"Though we travel the world over to find the beautiful,
we must carry it with us or we find it not."*

—Ralph Waldo Emerson

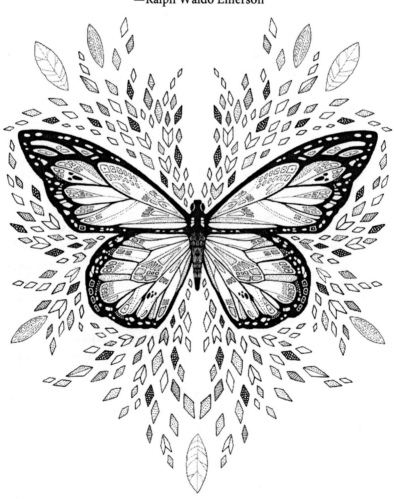

Chapter 23

Explore

Novelty can be exhilarating, yet terrifying. We are so intrigued by what is different, but we still often find ourselves sticking to the familiar, because it feels more comfortable.

Well, it turns out that embracing differences, seeking new experiences, and traveling to foreign places can make people happier, more open, more confident, and more adaptable to change. As Tim Bono, PhD, Lecturer in Psychology at Washington University in St. Louis, said in his TED Talk, "Learning How to Fail," "Don't let yourself get too comfortable, because that's when you stop growing."[1]

Gain Psychological Riches

In our modern, globalized world, it has become easier than ever to travel, whether to a distant destination around the world, or just to a neighboring city. And this is great news, because exposure to new environments is beneficial to personal development and growth. Fortunately, traveling is no longer reserved only for the elite. Varied and numerous transportation and accommodation methods have made travel more affordable than ever before. Also, tons of resources are available just searches away on the Internet to help you plan your itineraries, find the best deals, and budget your trip.

A study on students who participated in home-stay programs overseas (i.e., study-abroad programs where students live with host families) found that the experience significantly increased students' appreciation and understanding of their host country, culture, and language.[2] The experience also helped the students to gain a more global perspective on the world—a positive change that facilitates personal growth and makes one feel more connected to the world at large.

Especially at a time when many of us have become disconnected from our world—making us less aware of the impacts of our daily decisions—the ability to connect with people in other cities around the world and see them simply as our neighbors is extremely important in cultivating a sense of unity, harmony, and common purpose.

In our rapidly evolving world, research has shown that many people today have poor coping skills when confronting personal, social, and global changes.[3] How can we become more adaptable to change? Unfortunately, this is easier said than done; it is not a lesson that can be fully learned within classroom settings. Instead, it requires firsthand experiences facing, understanding, and adjusting to foreign environments and new situations.

Indeed, studies have found that living abroad also made students more agreeable, less neurotic, more confident, more open-minded, more independent, more stable in the face of uncertainty, and more adaptable to change.[4,5] It also made them less *ethnocentric* (less likely to perceive their own culture as superior), suggesting that travel can make people more understanding, more accepting, and less judgmental. So, it turns out that traveling can help us a lot more than just being something to check off on our bucket lists.

As Charles Darwin famously said, "It is not the strongest of the species that survives, nor the most intelligent that survives. It is the one that is most adaptable to change."

Get the Most Bang out of Your Buck

If you were given $500, what would you spend it on? A pair of expensive shoes? A winter coat? A coffee machine? The latest smartphone? To get the most satisfaction and happiness out of your money, you should think twice before making any of those decisions. A study found that *experiential purchases*, or purchases made with the intention of acquiring life experiences, made people happier than material purchases, or purchases made with the intention of obtaining material goods.[6] Examples of experiential purchases include eating a nice meal, going kayaking, getting a massage, going to see a movie, and exploring some place new. It is any purchase that involves *doing* rather than *having*. The researchers suggest that experiences make people happier because they are a more meaningful part of one's identity and contribute to strengthening social relationships.

A follow-up study found that, while the satisfaction people gained from experiences tended to increase over time, the satisfaction from material purchases tended to *decrease* over time.[7] Think about it: Experiential purchases give you wonderful memories to relive and reflect upon again and again, and they make much better stories to tell than the material goods you bought.

These findings are extremely important and relevant to the discussions in Part IV, "Beautify," and in Part V, "Style." While ridding ourselves of consumerism is impractical, shifting our values from quantity to quality, from the physical properties of a product to its rich history, and from material possessions to experiences will not only make us happier and healthier but will also make consumerism more sustainable.

Apparently, there is a similar dichotomy between experiential and possessive/materialistic attitudes when we travel, too. A recent study on nature tourism revealed that "appreciative" tourists had higher life satisfactions than "consumptive" tourists.[8] *Appreciative tourism* involves respectfully enjoying the experience of being in nature without altering it (i.e., *eco-tourism*). *Consumptive tourism*, however, is being more utilitarian, involving possession, extraction, or modification to the environment.[9]

While appreciative tourism emphasizes the culture and environment as a partner in the experience (e.g., wildlife watching), nonappreciative tourism stresses individuality and the exploitation of the environment (e.g., collecting artifacts and material possessions). Therefore, appreciative attitudes when traveling can increase life satisfaction by enhancing one's *connectedness to the environment*, while possessive/materialistic attitudes may elicit feelings of alienation instead.[10]

Transformative Traveling

People travel and explore all the time, but how do you make the most of the experience? Many people visit places to mark them off their bucket lists, but have they truly *been* there if they were there only to take photos of monuments and landscapes? Two people can go to the same city for the same duration but have vastly different experiences, depending on their attitudes. While each of us travels for our own reasons and interests, here are my personal tips on how to make the most of any traveling experience:

- Be a respectful traveler, and do some background research before you go somewhere new. What are its cultural customs? Dress code? Social etiquette? How do you say "Hello" and "Thank you" in their language?

- Be open-minded. Try things you have never tried before, eat food you have never had before, befriend people from the local community, and seek out hidden gems unknown to typical tourists.

- Seek to understand why things are the way they are, rather than making comparisons or judgments.

- Learn as much as you can, be observant, and immerse yourself into the local scene and culture, rather than just sticking to what is familiar to you.

- Get comfortable with being uncomfortable. Traveling to places that are very different than you are used to can be daunting. However, as long as you explore safely while embracing uncertainty and novelty, you will enhance your understanding of the community and gain a broadened perspective on our world.

Your travel experience is unique to you, and what you get out of it depends on what you make of it. However, the one common necessity for *transformative traveling*—a traveling experience that facilitates personal growth and development—is to travel with an open, appreciative mind. Shannon O'Donnell, 2013 National Geographic Traveler of the Year, noted that, because the Internet has given us the chance to virtually tour a place before going there, it is easy to have preconceptions about what to expect. Instead, she suggests stripping oneself of all those expectations and maintaining a willingness to discover and learn. After all, we all collectively need to adopt this very same open mindset to fully appreciate our world as a whole and live toward better health and a greener future.

You Have the Power

A few summers ago, I volunteered at an orphanage in the countryside of Kenya. But as much as I wanted to positively impact the lives of the underprivileged children there, I wondered whether my presence would make a difference. Would they be receptive to me as a stranger? Could I cultivate meaningful relationships with them without understanding Swahili?

On the third morning of my trip, my doubts vanished. When the children saw me walk through the school gates, they all lit up and started jumping around, collectively chanting, "Jambo! Jambo!" This happened every morning for the rest of my trip. Despite the language barrier, I was still able to develop intimate relationships with the kids simply by holding their hands, giving them attention and affection, and sharing moments of laughter with them. This made me realize that as human beings, we all share common desires for happiness and intimacy—regardless of where we come from or what languages we speak.

As you go about your daily life, remember how much impact you can have through your speech, body language, and actions. You may just be a stranger to the random people you encounter, but you can also choose to be a stranger with a positive impact. Maybe you will be that kind stranger who makes someone smile, or maybe you will be that thoughtful stranger who makes someone's day. A lot of positive changes in our neighborhoods, cities, countries, and even the world begin with just one person. And that person can be you.

It is easy to get discouraged by a lack of appreciation, affirmation, or acknowledgment from others when you try to do something selfless and thoughtful for someone else. But don't be, because your actions—what you personally control—are the most meaningful reflections of who you are (see also the "Recraft Your Mindset" section in Chapter 4). If you know that you are being the best person you can be, have faith in knowing that you have made the world a better place than it was.

Shannon O'Donnell took this concept of impact to a whole other level when she began Grassroots Volunteering, an organization that provides resources to empower travelers to connect to the causes and communities in the places they are traveling to. When you travel to a foreign place, being engulfed by unfamiliarity may make you feel vulnerable. However, keep in mind that you have the same power as you always do to impact people you encounter. Whether you take part in volunteer opportunities, support local social enterprises or businesses, befriend local citizens as a cultural exchange, or are simply a considerate and respectful traveler, making a positive difference in a completely foreign city can make your traveling experience much more meaningful to both you and the community you touch.

At the end of the day, just remember to keep a smile on your face, a universal sign of compassion and kindness that can elicit feelings of comfort and happiness in others—no matter their culture, religion, or place of origin.

Chapter Summary

Gain Psychological Riches

Traveling to foreign places—whether to a nearby town or to a city across the globe—that are very different than you are used to can be daunting and can make you feel uncomfortable. However, exposure to novel experiences can broaden your perspective on the world and make you more adaptable to change. These are some very valuable psychological resources you can gain only through life experiences.

Get the Most Bang out of Your Buck

To get the most bang for your buck, invest in more **experiential purchases** instead of material purchases. Because experiential purchases are more meaningful parts of your identity, they can make you happier and more satisfied, and even make consumerism more sustainable. Remember, "less is more," and focus on doing rather than having.

Transformative Traveling

We all travel for varying reasons and interests, but by traveling with an open mind and an **appreciative attitude,** we can make our experiences more insightful. Be a respectful traveler—learn the local cultural customs, seek to understand rather than to make judgments, immerse yourself into the local environment, and get comfortable with being uncomfortable.

You Have the Power

As discussed in Part I, "Smile," the best judgment of yourself is reflected in what you personally say and do. By becoming the best version of yourself, even when you go to a foreign place, you can be sure to not only make your trip a life-changing experience but also positively influence the community you touch.

Chapter 24

Thrive

Whenever I look at satellite photos of Earth, it always amazes me how minuscule each of us is. Isn't it shocking to know how much humans have transformed entire landscapes on our planet?

Unfortunately, we are currently entering what scientists are calling the *sixth mass extinction* (mass extinctions have occurred only five times in the past 540 million years), which is characterized by an exceptionally rapid loss of biodiversity.[11] While the extinction of species naturally occurs in the wild, the *amount* that has occurred over the past century—most attributed to human activity—has driven this natural rate to unnatural, alarming levels. Even under very conservative measures, the average rate of species loss over the last century has been estimated to be 100 times higher than the "background" rate.[12] Perhaps it is a disconnect between humans and nature—coupled with a lack of understanding—that created such a deleterious and dramatic consequence. But this should be a wake-up call to us all. Now that we know better, it is up to us to implement immediate change, as "the window of opportunity [for intensified conservation efforts] is rapidly closing."[13]

It seems that we have underestimated the powers and complexities of nature—the powers that have been evolving for millions of years to govern, balance, and maintain our planet's ecosystems. It is time we use lessons learned from our past to reshape and rebuild a healthier future for us all. We are collectively very impactful, but that power only begins with our choices as individuals. There is just so much meaning to discover behind every decision we make, if only we find it in ourselves the curiosity and passion to do so. From here on out, we need to combine our knowledge and power to work in *harmony* with our world—not against it.

I believe that people are inherently good, and that by shifting our stance from insensitivity to mindfulness and from division to unity, we will all have a better chance to *thrive together*.

Add Context to Poetry

If we focus only on the end results—how a shirt looks, if a shampoo will make our hair shinier, how much our salaries are, or how tasty something is—we will already be failing the test of sustainability. Focusing purely on the outcome dismisses the most important part of the equation: the process of the journey itself.

Our five senses may make our lives poetic, but from here on out, we need to dig deeper and build context around that poetry. We need to understand where things come from, how things are made, who made them, what conditions they were made in, and what impact they have on people and the environment.

By unraveling the stories behind all of the food and products we consume, we can transform our empty purchases into meaningful experiences. By shifting our focus away from end results to the processes within each of our own lives, we can begin to truly live and savor our moments in time.

As discussed in Part I, "Smile," happiness is not about achieving something or acquiring some physical good at one point in time. It is about crafting an ongoing positive attitude and way of living that will push us to always find the silver lining in the cloud and discover a sense of purpose in everything we do.

No More Lost in Translation

Now comes the time when you turn your desires and values into action. By getting in touch with the stories behind everything you support, you will gain a clearer understanding of how your daily decisions align with your values. By choosing to live positively, to take care of your body so you can function at your maximum potential, to eat nutritious food grown in healthful ways, to shop consciously, to support responsible practices, and to explore our world with a purpose, you will be well on your way to gaining true wealth and living a fulfilling life.

Of course, there is no easy way to change lifestyle habits. No one is perfect, but every little decision counts. No matter what long-term changes you are trying to achieve, remember that they all begin first with you becoming more aware of your actions (see also Chapter 3). You can achieve this by setting up frequent reminders for yourself to be more aware of what you are doing. Then, you will need to use your knowledge to help you make more informed, healthier choices.

While this book focuses on how you can live healthier by making more conscious everyday decisions, there are definitely other ways for us to address the many social and environmental issues that threaten our welfare today. One other way we can do this is through voting for what we believe in. We need to support laws that aim to keep us from getting sick in the first place, such as those that push for stricter regulations, more preventative care, and more transparency in complex industries. We also need to fight for policies that will ensure we keep pollution to a minimum, support organizations working to clean up the mess we have already created, and encourage urban development projects that green our cities.

Of course, using politics for positive social and environmental change is extremely complex and deserves much more attention, knowledge, and research than I have currently provided in this brief note. But just remember that, if you want to fight for something (which I highly encourage), always look for objective, well-supported information and hear both sides of the same argument in an open-minded way before making your personal conclusions and voicing your opinions.

Finally, we all know the power of word of mouth. Globalization and technology have made it so easy to spread information. Together, we can use this to our advantage. The path to a healthier, more sustainable world based on our daily decisions depends on *all* of us collectively recrafting our lifestyles.

Therefore, I need your help in sharing this challenge for all of us to broaden our definitions of "healthy" and to live a more positive, mindful lifestyle. To do so, share what you have discovered on holistic health through this book, your own research, or your personal life experiences (using #ThriveTheBook) so we can connect with one another, build a community, and generate momentum together to drive impactful changes on a global scale.

If You Are Human, You Are an Environmentalist

While I have attempted to make this healthy lifestyle guide as comprehensive and well supported as possible, I acknowledge that it is not perfect, nor do I have the answers to everything. Additionally, not everything we know right now, even conclusions from research studies, is the absolute truth. Every new scientific finding, every technological breakthrough, and every natural change in our ecosystem can alter our current understanding of the world. Therefore, I strongly encourage you to stay open-minded and thirsty for knowledge. Despite all of these uncertainties and potential circumstantial changes, however, our priorities should always remain the same: we must always put our health and the health of our entire planet first.

Meanwhile, instead of relying on any one particular study to make our lifestyle choices, we need to take a step back and look at everything in a more holistic manner. In a way, writing this book was like conducting a massive and broad, qualitative, meta-analysis of healthy living. And what I have learned from my research all seems to support the following conclusion made in Eleonora Gullone's review on the various literature discussing biophilia:

> Although more research is required so that specific conclusions can be made, there is substantial evidence to suggest that, as a species, our modern lifestyle may have strayed too far from that to which we have adapted.[14]

To live sustainably, we need to first get back in touch with our natural survival instincts and understand what our minds, bodies, and natural environments need in order to function healthily. We must then use this knowledge to reshape our thought processes, habits, and decisions. While each of us individually is just one person, all of our individual, everyday choices add up to create the massive impact that the human population has on our planet as a whole. It is time to broaden the concept of what we call home, and it is time to unite our world with our common purpose. In this journey toward a thriving you and a thriving planet, we are all in it together.

As it comes time for me to wrap up this book, it is also time for me to share the revelation I came to from piecing together the puzzle of good health and world sustainability:

> We are all one interconnected world, and we can no longer view the world as humans versus nature. Instead, there is just nature, of which we are an amazingly impactful part of. When we hurt our environment, we just end up hurting ourselves. What we create may be considered "artificial" and therefore not a part of "nature," but we as humans are a part of nature (because yes, we are a species of animal). The same laws that govern our planet's health are the same laws that govern ours. We do not function on natural gas, electricity, and fuel. We are not machines or robots. Instead, we thrive on clean air, clean water, sunlight, and nutritious and diverse food sources, just like our planet does. To threaten any of our necessities of life is to threaten our own well-being. Therefore, so long as we are human, we must also be environmentalists. Only when we are able to see the world as our home and judge our health holistically in conjunction with the health of our natural ecosystems will we understand how caring for ourselves is caring for our planet, and that caring for our planet is caring for ourselves.

Going Full Circle

Do you want to breathe fresh air, drink clean water, and swim in uncontaminated lakes, rivers, and oceans? Would you like to eat food that's tasty and nutritious, use lotion that is moisturizing and nontoxic, and wear clothing that will make you look and feel good? Do you want to live a long, healthy, happy, and fulfilling life?

Do you want to help reduce conflict, labor abuse, animal abuse, unfair wages, and unsafe working conditions for workers and farmers? Do you want to help work toward social and environmental justice and world sustainability? Do you want to help make the world a better place for you, your loved ones, your neighbors, and all of the other cohabitants of our planet?

Well, my dear neighbor, just start by truly caring for yourself and recrafting your life. If you are ready for this journey, let us *thrive* together on our thriving planet.

Chapter Summary

Add Context to Poetry

Our five senses may make our lives poetic, but it's time to add context to our poetry. By shedding light on the production processes of our consumer goods rather than judging them solely based on their physical properties, and by valuing the journey of our own lives rather than only living for the outcomes, we will be able to feel more engaged with our lives and reconnect with our world as one whole.

No More Lost in Translation

In any long-term lifestyle change, **awareness** and **understanding** must come first. I hope *Thrive* has helped you to gain an awareness of the impacts your choices can have, and I hope it has also deepened your understanding of your mind, body, and natural environment. Now, it is up to you to take action and translate your motivations into reality.

If You Are Human, You Are an Environmentalist

We are not exempt from the laws that govern the health of nature. We, too, need clean waters, unpolluted air, sunlight, and diverse, nutritious food sources in order to thrive. Therefore, so long as we are human, we must also be environmentalists. By taking a broader perspective of health (i.e., one that encompasses the health of our minds, bodies, and collective environment), we will all have a better chance to thrive together.

Going Full Circle

The human population is extremely impactful collectively, but that power only begins with the individual. By each of us cultivating a healthier mindset, adopting healthier habits, and making healthier daily decisions, we can turn our collective power into a force for good.

Part References

1   Bono, T. (2014) *Learning how to fail.* Speech presented at TedTalk, St. Louis.

2   Hansel, B., & Grove, N. (1986). International student exchange programs— Are the educational benefits real? *NASSP Bulletin, 70*(487), 84-90.

3   Seaward, B. L. (2013). *Managing stress: Principles and strategies for health and well-being.* Sudbury, MA: Jones and Bartlett.

4   Thomlison, T. D. (1991). Effects of a study-abroad program on university students: Toward a predictive theory of intercultural contact. *ERIC # ED 332 629.*

5   Zimmermann, J., & Neyer, F. J. (2013). Do we become a different person when hitting the road? Personality development of sojourners. *Journal of Personality and Social Psychology, 105*(3), 515-530.

6   Boven, L. V., & Gilovich, T. (2003). To do or to have? That is the question. *Journal of Personality and Social Psychology, 85*(6), 1193-1202.

7   Carter, T. J., & Gilovich, T. (2010). The relative relativity of material and experiential purchases. *Journal of Personality and Social Psychology, 98*(1), 146-159.

8   Bimonte, S., & Faralla, V. (2013). Happiness and outdoor vacations: Appreciative versus consumptive tourists. *Journal of Travel Research, 54*(2), 179-192.

9   Dunlap, R. E., & Hefferman, R. B. (1975). Outdoor recreation and environmental concern: An empirical examination. *Rural Sociology, 401*(1), 18-30.

10 Bimonte, S., & Faralla, V. (2013). Happiness and outdoor vacations: Appreciative versus consumptive tourists. *Journal of Travel Research, 54*(2), 179-192.

11 Ceballos, G., Ehrlich, P. R., Barnosky, A. D., Garcia, A., Pringle, R. M., & Palmer, T. M. (2015). Accelerated modern human-induced species losses: Entering the sixth mass extinction. *Science Advances, 1*(5), e1400253.

12 Ceballos, G., Ehrlich, P. R., Barnosky, A. D., Garcia, A., Pringle, R. M., & Palmer, T. M. (2015). Accelerated modern human-induced species losses: Entering the sixth mass extinction. *Science Advances, 1*(5), e1400253.

13 Ceballos, G., Ehrlich, P. R., Barnosky, A. D., Garcia, A., Pringle, R. M., & Palmer, T. M. (2015). Accelerated modern human-induced species losses: Entering the sixth mass extinction. *Science Advances, 1*(5), e1400253.

14 Gullone, E. (2000). The biophilia hypothesis and life in the 21st century: Increasing mental health or increasing pathology? *Journal of Happiness Studies, 1*(3), 293-322.

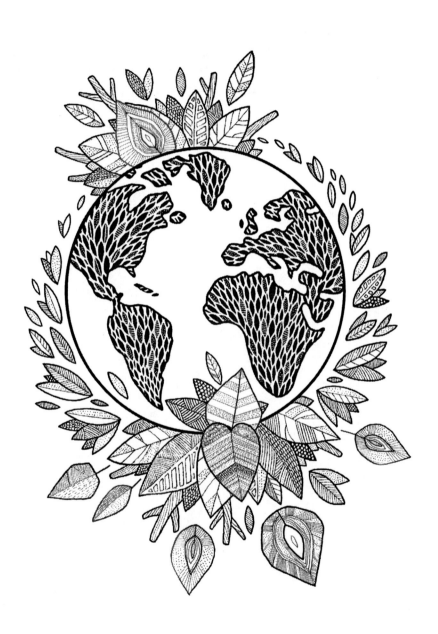

Closing Note

If you have completed this book, I want to sincerely thank you. Your time, interest, and support mean the world to me, and I am eternally grateful to have been able to touch your life. I hope you were able to gain something of value from the reading, and I wish you the best of luck with your journey toward better health and true wealth. May your life be filled with love, wisdom, blessings, meaningful riches, good health, and lots of healthy choices!

—K. Chayne

Acknowledgments

Words cannot begin to describe how thankful I am for every learning experience I've had in my life and every person I was lucky enough to have met.

My family: Thank you for *always* believing in me and unconditionally supporting everything I do. Thank you for the life-changing opportunities you have provided me with, and thank you for encouraging me to chase after my dreams.

Madalyn Stone: Thank you for being the most amazing editor I could have asked for. I could not have done this without your insightful, expert, and constructive feedback!

Todd Larson: Thank you for your assistance polishing *Thrive*. Your impeccable attention to detail and your thoughtful advice are highly appreciated.

Ashley Hudson and Krystal Huang: Thank you for being there for every step of *Thrive's* development. You were an integral part of this journey.

To all my teachers and professors at Taipei American School (TAS) and Washington University in St. Louis (WUSTL): Thank you for being a part of my life-changing educational journey, and thank you for helping to shape who I am and what I know today.

I would also like to thank the following people who have been huge inspirations to me, people from whom I was lucky enough to have learned much throughout my writing process, people who have contributed to this book with their expert knowledge or artistic talent, and people who have wholeheartedly supported me through it all (in alphabetical order):

Dan Barber, chef and co-owner of Blue Hill; Nicole Bell, yoga instructor; Tim Bono, PhD, professor at WUSTL; Mark Browne, PhD, ecologist and ARC Senior Research Associate at the University of New South Wales; Janice Cantieri; Jennie Chang; Kevin Chang; Molly Chester, co-owner of Apricot Lane Farms; Jamie Cote, independent health coach; Julifer Day, fitness trainer and creator of "Day by Day Training"; Mikala Evans; Brent Hiramoto; Victoria Horng; Krystal Huang, yoga instructor; Meilin Hyde; Michelle Jayne, yoga instructor; Nicole Kawamoto; Mara Keller; Madeline Kleiner; Liisa Kokkarinen; Stephanie Kuo; Faye Lessler of Sustaining.Life; Michael Lin; Jean Lin; Wendy Lin; Dan Long, educator at TAS; Renée Loux, culinary nutrition expert; William R. Lowry, PhD, professor at WUSTL; Jade Lu; Kasi Martin of The Peahen; Morgana Mellett, fitness trainer and founder of MOMO Momentum Training W/ Morgana LLC; Michael Merbaum, PhD, Professor at WUSTL; Esther Moon; Emily Ness; Shannon O'Donnell, 2013 National Geographic Traveler of the Year; Eleanor Pardini,

PhD, professor at WUSTL; Andrew Pierce, MS, RD, CSSD, CSCS; John Parks, PhD, professor at WUSTL; Elaine Partnow, developmental writing consultant; Ellen Passov, RDN, CDN; Francesca Rinaldi, professor at SDA Bocconi School of Management and Milano Fashion Institute; Laura Rosenberg, MS, RD, CDN, educator at Natural Gourmet Institute; Alex Rosenthal; Gavin Rutherford, cover and interiors illustrator; James Sawhill, PhD, professor at WUSTL; Helene Serignac, TV journalist; Kayleen St. John, MS, RD, educator at Natural Gourmet Institute; Michael Strube, PhD, professor at Washington University in St. Louis; Sharon Su; Spencer Tong; Chong Vue; Alden Wicker of EcoCult; Penny Wu; Xi Zhen Wu; Sandra Yeh, MD FAAD; Members of Ethical Writers Coalition.

Additional Resources

Smile More

- Diener, Ed, and Robert Biswas-Diener. *Happiness: Unlocking the Mysteries of Psychological Wealth*. Malden, Mass.: Wiley Blackwell, 2008.

- Hanson, Rick, Ph.D., with Richard Mendius, M.D. *Buddha's Brain: The Practical Neuroscience of Happiness, Love and Wisdom*. Oakland: New Harbinger Publications, 2009.

- Lyubomirsky, Sonja. *The How of Happiness: A New Approach to Getting the Life You Want*. New York: Penguin Press, 2008.

- Solomon, Andrew. *How the Worst Moments in our Lives Make Us Who We Are*. TED Talk, May 21, 2014.

- Watson, David L., and Roland G. Tharp.*Self-Directed Behavior: Self-Modification for Personal Adjustment*. Tenth edition. Belmont, Calif.: Wadsworth Publishing, 2013.

Revitalize More

- FitnessBlender.com, an online resource for workout videos for at-home exercise training.

- Youtube.com/Gaiam by Gaiam, an online resource for yoga videos for at-home exercise training.

Nourish More

- Anderson, Kip, and Keegan Kuhn. *Cowspiracy: The Sustainability Secret*. Directed by Kip Anderson and Keegan Kuhn. 2014. Los Angeles: A.U.M. Films, First Spark Media, 2014. DVD.

- Barber, Dan. *The Third Plate: Field Notes on the Future of Food*. New York: The Penguin Group, 2014.

- Choose My Plate (ChooseMyPlate.gov), an online resource by the United States Department of Agriculture on nutrition.

- Clement, Brian R. *Food is Medicine: The Scientific Evidence.* Summertown, Tenn.: Hippocrates Publications, 2012.

- EatWild.com, an international online directory of pasture-based farms.

- Haas, Elson M., and Buck Levin. *Staying Healthy with Nutrition: The Complete Guide to Diet and Nutritional Medicine.* Berkeley: Celestial Arts, 2006.

- Local Harvest (LocalHarvest.org), an online resource for locating nearby farms and farmers' markets.

- Minger, Denise. *Death by Food Pyramid: How Shoddy Science, Sketchy Politics and Shady Special Interests Have Conspired to Ruin the Health of America.* First Edition. Malibu, Calif.: Primal Blueprint Publishing, 2014.

- Monterey Bay Aquarium Seafood Watch (SeafoodWatch.org), an online resource for finding sustainable seafood.

- Natural Gourmet Institute (NaturalGourmetInstitute.com) a school of sustainable gourmet cooking.

- Pollan, Michael. *The Omnivore's Dilemma.* New York: Penguin Group, 2006.

- RaRa (wearerara.com), a magazine on sustainable cooking.

- Rockefeller, Susan Cohn. *Food for Thought, Food for Life.* Directed by Susan Cohn Rockefeller. 2015.

- Seasonal Food Guide (SustainableTable.org/SeasonalFoodGuide), an online seasonal food guide.

Beautify More

- Cosmetics Info (CosmeticsInfo.org), an online resource on self-care products.

Style More

- Clement, Anna Maria, and Brian R. Clement. *Killer Clothes: How Seemingly Innocent Clothing Choices Endanger Your Health—and How to Protect Yourself!* Summertown, Tenn.: Hipprocrates Publications, 2011.

- Fashion Revolution (FashionRevolution.org), an organization dedicated to making the fashion industry more sustainable.

- Fletcher, Kate. *Sustainable Fashion and Textiles: Design journeys*. London: Earthscan, 2008.

- Morgan, Andrew. *The True Cost*. Directed by Andrew Morgan. 2015. A documentary on the fashion industry's social and environmental impacts.

- Rinaldi, Francesca Romana, and Salvo Testa. *The Responsible Fashion Company: Integrating Ethics and Aesthetics in the Supply Chain*. Sheffield: Greenleaf Publishing, 2014.

- Styles, Ruth. *Ecologist Guide to Fashion*. Lewes, U.K.: The Ivy Press, 2014.

- The Zady Chronicle (Zady.com/features), a blog on sustainable fashion by Zady.

Transform More and More

- Ethical Writers Co. (EthicalWriters.co), lifestyle resources by writers, journalists, and bloggers of the EWC.

- *Eluxe*, a lifestyle magazine.

- Environmental Working Group (ewg.org), an organization dedicated to protecting human health and the environment.

- *Kinfolk*, a lifestyle magazine.

- MindBodyGreen.com, an online lifestyle publication.

- Moment For Action (MomentForAction.org), an online resource for people interested in making a difference on climate change.

- Natural Resources Defense Council (nrdc.org), an environmental action group with the latest environmental news and other general eco-lifestyle resources.

- O'Donnell, Shannon. *The Volunteer Traveler's Handbook: How to Find Ethical and Sustainable International Volunteer Opportunities*. Orlando, Fla.: Full Flight Press, 2012.

- *Remarkable*, a lifestyle magazine.

- *Thoughtfully* (thoughtfullymag.com), a lifestyle magazine of thoughtful and intentional living.

- Well + Good (wellandgood.com), an online lifestyle publication.

- Youtube.com/theHealthcareTriage, an online resource for evidence-based information on healthcare by Dr. Aaron Carroll

Index

D

farmers 103, 104, 108-111, 113, 114, 170, 222
  and agrobiodiversity 119
  and fair trade 193
  and toxic chemicals 197
  suicides of 108
  working conditions of 166, 222
farmers' markets 103, 119, 122, 232
farming 55, 102-103, 104, 124
  and biodiversity 119, 121
  biodynamic 109
  factory farming 110-111
  Indonesian 108
  sustainable 103
  organic 104, 105, 108, 109
fashion 165-170, 171
  cycle of 167
  diversity in 188
  eco-fashion 169, 194
  environmental hazards of 166-167
  environmental impacts of 169, 189
  "fast fashion" 167, 171, 183
  marketing stataements 177, 191
  Rent the Runway (fashion rental company) 184
  "slow fashion" 167-168, 171, 183
  "sustainable fashion" 183-189, 190
fashion brands:
  Benetton 167
  Dior 177
  Dolce & Gabbana 177
  H&M 167, 168
  Hermès 177
  Levi's 501 jeans 179
  Primark 167
  Zara 167
fashion brands (eco-conscious):
  Patagonia 176, 192-193
  People Tree 192

United by Blue 193
  Zady 193
fat 43
fats 86, 88, 95, 96
  and obesity 87
  full-fat paradox 87
  saturated fats 87
  trans fats 87, 95, 96
  unsaturated fats 87
fatigue 74, 75, 147, 180
  in muscles 178
fear 12, 60
feet 72, 79
fertility 179
fertilizers 109
fetus 139, 142, 145
fiber 86, 95, 96, 98, 101
  and digestion 98
  organic 193
  Also see **synthetic fibers**
Firth, Livia 172
fish see **seafood**
fishing see **water**
fitness 42-53, 54, 56, 59
  cardiorespiratory 51-52
  fitness trainer 60
5 Gyres Organization 172
flax:
  dew-retted 185, 189
  organic 185, 189
Fletcher, Kate 189
flexibility 14
  of the body 42, 43-50, 54
Flint, Michigan 142-143
Flint River 142-143
flowers 3, 155
  daisies 116
  pollination of 116
  sunflowers 115-116
flu (influenza) 16
food 55, 85, 86-92, 93, 95-98, 102-112, 111-112, 126-127
  and chemical interactions 87, 93, 97, 101

through positive thinking 1
ingredients 89-90, 93, 142-151,
    152
    disclosure of 197, 198
    nontoxic 156, 197
    sustainable 154
injury 56
    and alcohol 100
injustice 34
insects 104
    bees 116
    mosquitoes 173
insecticides see **chemicals**
insomnia 78
inspiration 10, 11, 17, 20
Instagram 32
Institute of Medicine 106
insulation 197, 200
International Joint Commission
    143
Internet:
    for product research 155, 194
    for travel resources 212, 215
    SeafoodWatch.org 112
interpretation of situations 8-9,
    11
intimacy 28
introspection 22
Inuit 119
invasive species 202
iron:
    heme iron 97
    nonheme iron 97
isolation 73
Italy 123
    Italian cuisine 123, 126

J

Japan 91, 119, 123
    hara hachi bu 91
    Okinawa 91
Jayne, Michelle (yoga instructor)
    15

jobs 24-25, 28, 30-31
jogging 52
Johnson, Bea 201, 202
joints 44-50
journaling 75, 77, 80
journeys:
    of clothing 166, 169, 170
    of food 108, 109
    of life 6, 28, 222, 223
    of sustainability 219
joy 12
judgment:
    impaired 99
    of appearance 51
    of food 102-103, 128
    of products 168, 171, 183, 223
    of others 213
    of our health 221
    of ourselves 215, 217
    of the world 215, 217
junk food 23, 43, 90, 91, 93, 95-96
    as a drug 96, 101
    cakes 95
    candy 95
    cookies 95, 96
    harmfulness 96, 101

K

Kazakhstan 185
Kenya 119, 215
kidneys 89, 125, 139, 145, 180
    kidney disease 95, 96
kindness 26, 29, 215, 216
knees 48, 62, 63, 65, 66, 68, 71, 79

L

labels, fashion:
    "antistatic" 177
    B Corp 193
    Ecolabel by the European Union
    193
    "ethical" 192, 195

About the Author

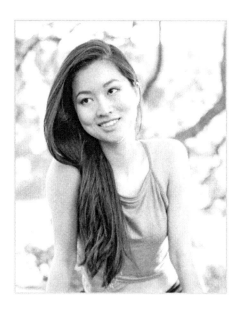

Kamea Chayne is a graduate of Washington University in St. Louis, where she studied psychology, environmental studies, and marketing. She is passionate about eco-design, mind-body wellness, and transformative traveling.

Through her multidisciplinary studies and her multicultural background, she developed a particular interest in the relationship between human health and world sustainability—an interest that eventually led her to write her debut non-fiction book, *Thrive*. By proposing a broadened perspective on health—one that encompasses the health of the mind, body, and our collective environment—Chayne hopes to empower her readers to cultivate meaning and create sustainability in all areas of life.

www.KChayne.com

CPSIA information can be obtained
at www.ICGtesting.com
Printed in the USA
FSOW02n1828010616
21053FS